Animal-assisted Interventions

Recognizing and Mitigating Potential Welfare Challenges

Animal-assisted Interventions

Recognizing and Mitigating Potential Welfare Challenges

Lori R. Kogan, PhD
Colorado State University, USA

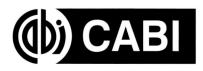

CABI is a trading name of CAB International

CABI
Nosworthy Way
Wallingford
Oxfordshire OX10 8DE
UK

CABI
200 Portland Street
Boston, MA
02114
USA

Tel: +44 (0)1491 832111
E-mail: info@cabi.org
Website: www.cabi.org

T: +1 (617)682-9015
E-mail: cabi-nao@cabi.org

The views expressed in this publication are those of the author(s) and do not necessarily represent those of, and should not be attributed to, CAB International (CABI). Any images, figures and tables not otherwise attributed are the author(s)' own. References to internet websites (URLs) were accurate at the time of writing. CAB International and, where different, the copyright owner shall not be liable for technical or other errors or omissions contained herein. The information is supplied without obligation and on the understanding that any person who acts upon it, or otherwise changes their position in reliance thereon, does so entirely at their own risk. Information supplied is neither intended nor implied to be a substitute for professional advice. The reader/user accepts all risks and responsibility for losses, damages, costs and other consequences resulting directly or indirectly from using this information.

CABI's Terms and Conditions, including its full disclaimer, may be found at https://www.cabi.org/terms-and-conditions/.

A catalogue record for this book is available from the British Library, London, UK.

ISBN-13: 9781800622593 (paperback)
         9781800622609 (ePDF)
         9781800622616 (ePub)

DOI: 10.1079/ 9781800622616.0000

Commissioning Editor: Alexandra Lainsbury
Editorial Assistant: Lauren Davies
Production Editor: Shankari Wilford

Typeset by Exeter Premedia Services Pvt Ltd, Chennai, India
Printed and bound in the USA by Integrated Books International, Dulles, Virginia

Contents

Part 6: Adults

Contributors

Patti Anderson, MEd, Doggone Good Coaching, LLC, Plymouth, Minnesota, USA. Email: Siberpa@aol.com

Ursula A. Aragunde Kohl, PsyD, Universidad Ana G. Méndez, Gurabo Campus, Gurabo, Puerto Rico. Email: Aragundeu1@uagm.edu

Nicky Barendrecht-Jenken, MSc, Stichting AAI-maatje, Gouda, the Netherlands. Email: Info@aai-maatje.nl

Darlene Blackman, Marin Humane, Novato, California, USA. Email: Dblackman@marinhumane.org

Eileen Bona, MEd, Dreamcatcher Nature Assisted Therapy, Ardrossan, Alberta, Canada. Email: Eileen@dreamcatcherassociation.com

Donna Clarke, LCPC, NCC, BC-TMH, CIMHP, CCTP-II, CGP, C-DBT, Linganore Counseling and Wellness, LLC, New Market, Maryland, USA. Email: Donnac42086@gmail.com

Linda Chassman Craddock, PhD, LMFT, CAAP, C-AAIS, Animal Assisted Therapy Programs of Colorado, Arvada, Colorado, USA. Email: Lchassman@aatpc.org

Yvonne Eaton-Stull, DSW, MSW, LCSW, Slippery Rock University, Slippery Rock, Pennsylvania, USA. Email: yvonne.eaton-stull@sru.edu

Nina Ekholm Fry, MSSc., CCTP, Institute for Human-Animal Connection, University of Denver, Denver, Colorado, USA. Email: Nina.ekholm-fry@du.edu

Aubrey H. Fine, PhD, California State Polytechnic University, Pomona, California, USA. Email: Ahfine@gmail.com

Cynnie Foss, University of Washington Medical Center, Seattle, Washington, USA. Email: Fossc@uw.edu

Angela Fournier, PhD, LP, Bemidji State University, Bemidji, Minnesota, USA. Email: Angela.Fournier@bemidjistate.edu

Megan French, BS, Eagle Vista Ranch, Bemidji, Minnesota, USA. Email: mnfrench27@gmail.com

Lisa-Maria Glenk, MSc, PhD Messerli Research Institute (Comparative Medicine) and University College for Agricultural and Environmental Pedagogy, Vienna, Austria. Email: Lisa.molecular@gmail.com

Temple Grandin, PhD, Department of Animal Science, Colorado State University, Fort Collins, Colorado, USA. Email: templegrandincattle@gmail.com

Susan D. Greenbaum, LCSW, RxCanines – Therapeutic Intervention Dogs, Milford, New Jersey, USA. Email: barkinghills@gmail.com

Taylor Chastain Griffin, PhD, Pet Partners, Association of Animal-Assisted Intervention Professionals (AAAIP), Bellevue, Washington, USA. Email: Taylorc@petpartners.org

Joy R. Hanson, BA (Pschology), MA (Clinical Mental Health Counseling) in progress, Colorado Christian University, Lakewood, Colorado, USA. Email: hansonjoy1972@gmail.com

Terri Hlava, PhD, Human Animal Bond In Teaching and Therapies (H.A.B.I.T.A.T.), School of Social Transformation, Arizona State University, Tempe, Arizona, USA. Email: Thlava@asu.edu

Ann R. Howie, CCA, CCFT, LICSW, ACSW, Human-Animal Solutions, PLLC, Olympia, Washington, USA. Email: Humananimalsolutions@comcast.net

Batya G. Jaffe, PhD, AAT, Wurzweiler School of Social Work, Yeshiva University, New York, USA. Email: Bjaffe2@mail.yu.edu

Amy Johnson, EdD, MA, MAT, LPC, CPDT-KA, UW-AAB, Oakland University, Rochester, Michigan, USA. Email: dramyjohnsonlpc@gmail.com

Suzanne M. Kapral, MS, The Lands at Hillside Farms, Shavertown, Pennsylvania, USA. Email: Suzanne@thelandsathillsidefarms.org

Jean Kirnan, PhD, PHR, The College of New Jersey, Ewing Township, New Jersey, USA. Email: Jkirnan@tcnj.edu

Veronica Lac, LPC, PhD, The HERD Institute, Orlando, Florida, USA. Email: veronica@herdinstitute.com

Elizabeth A. Letson, MS, LPCC, Owner and CEO, Eagle Vista Ranch & Wellness Center, Bemidji, Minnesota, USA; Adjunct Psychology Faculty, Bemidji State University, Bemidji, Minnesota, USA. Email: eaglevistaranch@gmail.com

Helen Lewis, PhD, SFHEA, FCCT, Department of Education and Childhood Studies, Swansea University, Swansea, Wales, UK. Email: Helen.e.lewis@swansea.ac.uk

Kirsty MacQueen, MA, ABTC-ATI, CAEBS, Therapawsitive CIC, Glasgow, Scotland, UK. Email: Kirstykmq@gmail.com

Arieahn Matamonasa-Bennett, PhD, Licensed Psychologist and equine-assisted psychotherapy (EAP) practitioner, Chicago, Illinois, USA. Email: amatamo1@depaul.edu

Angela M. Moe, PhD, Director of Therapy Dog Clinic, Department of Sociology, Western Michigan University, Kalamazoo, Michigan, USA. Email: Angie.moe@wmich.edu

Julie Ann Nettifee, RVT, MS, VTS (Neurology), NC State College of Veterinary Medicine, Raleigh, North Carolina, USA. Email: Janettif2@gmail.com

Zenithson Ng, DVM, MS, Dipl ABVP, University of Tennessee College of Veterinary Medicine, Knoxville, Tennessee, USA. Email: zng@utk.edu

Brittany Panus, PLPC, NCC, West Lane Elementary, Jackson, Missouri, USA. Email: Brittanylp92@gmail.com

B. Caitlin Peters, PhD, OTR/L, Temple Grandin Equine Center, Colorado State University, Fort Collins, Colorado, USA. Email: caiti.peters@colostate.edu

Laura Poleshuck, PhD, OTD, OTR/L, Nazareth University, Rochester, New York, USA. Email: Lpolesh3@naz.edu

Missy Reed, MSEd, MT-BC, Nazareth University, Rochester, New York, USA. Email: mreed8@naz.edu

Elizabeth Ruegg, MSW, Saint Leo University, St. Leo, Florida, USA. Email: Elizabeth.ruegg@saintleo.edu

Brenda Rynders, MSc, Animal Hospital of Sebastopol and Sheepy Hollow Sanctuary, Sebastopol, California, USA. Email: Brendalu2527@gmail.com

Sarah Schlote, MA, RP, CCC, SEP, EQUUSOMA® Horse–Human Trauma Recovery, Guelph, Ontario, Canada. Email: info@equusoma.com

Shira Smilovici, PhD, Prepa ibero and Clínica de Psicoterapia Asistida por Animales (CLIPA) AAT, Lerma, Mexico. Email: sc.shira@gmail.com

Ashley Thompson, certified teacher, MAT, West Belmar Elementary School, Wall Township, New Jersey, USA. Email: athompson@wallpublicschools.org

Anna van den Berg, credentials unknown, Reading Education Assistance Dogs (READ), Salt Lake City, Utah, USA. Email: info@readnederland.nl

Risë VanFleet, PhD, RPT-S, CDBC, CAEBI, International Institute for Animal Assisted Play Therapy®, Boiling Springs, Pennsylvania, USA. Email: Rise@risevanfleet.com

Melissa Y. Winkle, OTR/L, FAOTA, CPDT-KA, Dogwood Therapy Services Inc., Albuquerque, NM, USA. Email: Melissa@dogwoodtherapy.com

Katrina Winsor, MS, C-AAIS, CPDT-KA, CBCC-KA, The New Interdisciplinary School, Yaphank, New York, USA. Email: Katrinaw@niskids.org

Foreword

When a psychologist and veterinarian are called upon to advocate for animal welfare in animal-assisted interventions (AAIs), we answer. We come to this field with distinctly different training and experience. As a licensed psychologist, I (Aubrey) am trained to look at the process from the human side of this equation, but with my extensive experience in the field, I have always acted as an animal welfare advocate. As a veterinarian, I (Zenny) am very cognizant of the unique needs of the animals. We urge all clinicians to consider both ends of the leash when providing AAI and are excited for this much-needed applied text—written for those who want to ensure that they are protecting and promoting the welfare of their animal partners when providing AAIs.

A Psychologist's Perspective

When I began my work in the field of AAI, there was not only a dearth of useful information about how to apply AAIs, but also little to no concern about the welfare of therapy animals. Although well intended, most of the clinical emphasis was focused on the human benefits from the relationship. That is not to say that people were not concerned about therapy animal well-being, but the impetus of the work was largely centered on the benefits for humans.

It is difficult for me to realize that it has been 50 years since I first started to work with children alongside animals. Yet, I recognized many years ago that it was my responsibility to ensure the well-being of the animals with whom I worked. This position has not changed at all over the decades. I quickly realized that to do this work effectively and ethically, clinicians must be their animals' ambassadors. We must consider the ethical cost–benefit in applying AAIs, especially as it relates to preserving the integrity and well-being of therapy animals. Their lives and well-being must be our priority if we are going to do our jobs correctly. When addressing the animal's well-being, attention must be given, not only while they are working, but before and after their interactions.

Attention to animal welfare should begin early in a therapy animal's life. One must plan for the therapy animal's life trajectory of engagement, appreciating that the welfare considerations of a therapy animal change greatly as s/he ages. In essence, it is our ethical mandate to consider the animal's right to live naturally and thrive. As handlers, it is incumbent on us to accept our moral responsibility of being the animal's voice. In several articles we have written, we talk about the fact that "no longer should we think about what the animals can do for our clients, but rather what we as clinicians must do for the animals' well-being".

A focus on animal welfare strengthens a sustainable partnership. It is evident that teams built upon a foundation of animal well-being will be more successful in positively impacting clients within a therapeutic environment. In essence, prioritizing animal safety and wellness increases the efficacy of any interaction. When considering Mellor's five domains (i.e. nutrition, health, the physical environment, behavior, and mental state) (Mellor *et al.*, 2020), it is evident that clinicians must be trained to understand and be aware of these factors that impact an animal's quality of life. Additionally, handlers need to be aware of several other issues to protect their animals. They must have sufficient training in animal behavior to successfully implement welfare-based AAI protocols. More specifically, they need to be aware of their animals' natural behaviors, traits, personality, and ethology, as well as being mindful of species-specific welfare training practices. Handlers should also have a clear understanding of their animals' roles in AAI and be aware of the animals' interest in being involved. Animals should be given options and should have a safe retreat place to go when they need a break.

In essence, handlers must be aware of the many factors that can impact the stress of a therapy animal in the working environment. In an article that we authored in 2019, we discussed in detail that to understand welfare, one must consider how the handler, the participant, the environment, and the interaction all impact the animal; each of these dimensions has an impact on the animal's stress level. Becoming more aware of each of these factors can help prevent unnecessary stress. Handlers must have a good working relationship with their therapy animal partners. Personally, I suggest that the relationship between the animal and the handler needs to be seamless. I use the metaphor of dancing like Fred Astaire and Ginger Rogers as the way I've learned to work alongside therapy animals. We interact smoothly, which makes a greater impact on the overall outcome. Handlers must also recognize that not all animals can perform the expected jobs they are given. Handlers must consider what the job entails and select the animal that best suits that job description.

A prerequisite for an effective AAI practitioner is that s/he must be able to quickly identify when an animal is not comfortable and make immediate adjustments. Practitioners must be trained not only to apply AAIs in various settings, but to be conscious of how all accompanying factors involved in AAI impact their therapy partner. We have argued for years that successful AAIs require attention to all participants, human and animals, and we have a moral responsibility to ensure everyone's welfare. Pet Partners emphasizes this position the best with their acronym YAYABA—You Are Your Animal's Best Advocate. By taking this advice, handlers can navigate this process more versed in appreciating all the key elements of animal welfare and well-being.

A Veterinarian's Perspective

As a veterinarian, I aim to ensure the optimal physical and behavioral health for every animal I have the privilege of caring for, and therapy animals are no exception. Over the past two decades, I have seen handlers of all skill and knowledge levels and therapy animals of all varieties. Therapy animals are a very special "breed" and their owners, a very special type of clientele. I love working with the handlers who pride themselves on providing the best possible care for their co-partners. Not only do I benefit from the interactions I have with these pets, but I benefit from the inspiration these handlers bring me. I enjoy discovering why this person decided to enter the therapy animal world in the first place, the dynamics of their relationship with their co-partner, and what kinds of differences they make in people's lives. Conversations about these topics deepen my personal veterinarian–client–patient relationship and invigorate my passion for the work I am able to do for both humans and animals.

With regard to physical health, most of my therapy animal patients are generally in good health. More than just vaccines and dewormers, I enjoy challenging owners to take preventive health to the next level by offering tips and tricks that can make their pet's life even better yet. These recommendations vary from tailoring optimal nutrition, demonstrating physical fitness exercises, discussing joint supplements, or comparing the newest products for dental health. Owners are always keen to engage in these conversations to ensure their pets live the longest, healthiest lives possible. There are also situations where therapy animals may not be in pristine health and living with a chronic disease such as endocrine disorders, osteoarthritis, or heart disease. Although concerning, an animal being diagnosed with a disease does not automatically disqualify them from therapy work. It is my job as a veterinarian to determine whether the animal's clinical condition is properly managed and whether the welfare of the animal would be compromised as a result of therapy work.

With regard to behavioral health, I am quite impressed with the baseline behavior knowledge of most of my handlers. They are usually able to recognize their animal's body language and importantly, how their animal displays stress. The majority of therapy animals I meet in the clinic demonstrate exactly why they are a therapy animal. They are confident, friendly—and of course, adorable—creatures that immediately steal my heart. Although proper training and manners are critical in creating a good therapy animal, these are the qualities that cannot be taught or trained. When I think about the ideal therapy dog, I automatically reminisce about my first therapy dog, "Grace," who will forever be my soul dog. The reason she was the perfect therapy dog was not just because of her sweet face and obedient nature, but because she possessed the natural and unsolicited desire to say hello to each person, make gentle body contact with them, look at them in the eyes, and truly connect—making complete strangers feel like they were old friends. This ability does not require a high degree of friendliness and sociability, but does require the key element of trust. I believe that the immediate ability to trust others is unique to the most special therapy dogs. These are the dogs that wear their hearts on their sleeves and love fearlessly and unconditionally. These are the ones who were born to be therapy animals.

It is the dog who is distrusting and apprehensive of me that makes me question whether they were "born" to do this. Of course, the veterinary setting is a very stressful place, with strange scents and smells, and can understandably be an intimidating place for an animal. If, after my team and I have exhausted all the techniques we know to make friends with an animal, they are still untrusting and throwing out every stress signal in their vocabulary, I know it's time to dig a little deeper in determining the "goodness of fit" for their role as a therapy animal. I will assess the skill of the handler in reading their animal's body language and how proactive they are in advocating for their animal's welfare. I'll also tease out the reason they want to do therapy work. I have learned to appreciate that the most well-intentioned handlers may be resistant to accept that their animal may not be meant to be a therapy animal. Some handlers are blind to the fact that their animal simply does not want to do the work. This can be especially true when the animal does not display overt signs of aggression and obediently follows commands while consistently showing stress signals and a lack of enthusiasm for work.

I see this situation as similar to the ways in which well-intentioned parents push their children to engage in something they don't want to do. My parents forced me into piano lessons despite my resistance. Because I was given no choice in the matter, I reluctantly learned to play. While I was seemingly competent at it, I lacked the ability to excel to the level of concert pianist that my parents wanted because I lacked the passion and personal desire to do so. I look back upon this and appreciate my parents for trying to do what was good for me, but it was not who I was nor who I wanted to be. I sympathize with the animals who show me, through their body language, actions, and eyes, that they don't enjoy being therapy animals, but have an owner who enjoys being a therapy animal handler. These animals are pushed through training, pushed through therapy certification, and pushed through visits, yet this is not the vision of the human–animal bond. This is a difficult pill for some owners to swallow: not every animal is meant to be a therapy animal.

For those animals that are meant to be therapy animals, there is so much to be learned about their welfare during therapeutic work. We need to remember that not every human–animal interaction is positive and adverse events from these interactions can certainly occur. It is not just about petting animals. It is recognizing that every animal is a sentient being with unique wants and needs, and it is our duty to attend to those. The concrete needs such as protection from environmental hazards, providing water, and minimizing the risks of infectious disease are easy to address. Then there are less tangible needs such as ensuring their freedom to express normal behavior as well as the freedom to choose whether or not to engage—both of which are just as important to address. Assuring these needs are met requires a higher level of skill, intuition, and understanding of the animal. I believe that animals who truly love their work, the ones who truly trust all and love fearlessly—they live happier, longer, and healthier lives. The benefits of the human–animal bond occur when both human and animal mutually benefit, when both parties genuinely enjoy each other's company and find comfort and play in just being themselves. A complex, positive, symbiotic reaction happens both physiologically and emotionally when the right human–animal interaction occurs.

Our Concluding Remarks

There are so many critical lessons we must learn and teach others as we navigate the landscape of animal welfare in AAIs. To the undiscerning eye, therapy animal welfare may seem trivial when compared to other pressing animal welfare issues. However, a deeper look into the science of animal welfare within the context of the human–animal bond has the potential to ensure the best quality of life for every animal that interacts with a human being. As you read through the personal stories of these amazing professionals in the field, put yourself in the paws of the animal to appreciate how each animal truly thinks and feels. And recognize that good things happen when animal welfare is prioritized.

Aubrey H. Fine, PhD
California State Polytechnic University

Zenithson Ng, DVM, MS, Dipl ABVP
University of Tennessee College of Veterinary Medicine

Reference

Mellor, D.J., Beausoleil, N.J., Littlewood, K.E., McLean, A.N., McGreevy, P.D. *et al.* (2020) The 2020 five domains model: including human–animal interactions in assessments of animal welfare. *Animals* 10(10): 1870. DOI: 10.3390/ani10101870.

1 The Importance of Animal Welfare in Animal-assisted Services

MELISSA Y. WINKLE[1]* AND AMY JOHNSON[2]

[1]Dogwood Therapy Services Inc., Albuquerque, New Mexico, USA; [2]Oakland University, Rochester, Michigan, USA

Abstract

The domestication of animals by humans is grounded by a utilitarian approach. Most animal welfare and rights materials were written based on animals in agriculture, research, exhibition, and production. More progressive thinking has animals fulfilling the roles of family members and as helpers in healthcare and human services. While welfare currently describes the intrinsic value of animals, independent of humans, we may still be falling short based on how the *animal* experiences animal-assisted services (AAS). With this in mind, this chapter offers considerations for selection, preparation, training, and evaluation for AAS.

Introduction

Most animal-assisted services (AAS) providers have the very best of intentions when including animals in their session plans. For those who enjoy them, animals can elicit positive emotional states for humans via surges of oxytocin, dopamine, and serotonin. These interactions are often romanticized using human language to describe human perceptions in print, social media, television, and movies. But are the selected portrayals telling the full story? Back in the real world, many animals are having a different experience. We see dogs in classrooms with children laying on them and the dog guardian boasting of how "bombproof" the dog is with the kids, but the trained eye can see a dog who is shut down. The classroom rabbit that struggles to escape a child's tight embrace, only to be accidentally dropped or thrown in the struggle. Horses may have learned helplessness as they are tied to fence posts with short leads so teens can express their feelings by painting on them. We hear of animals being unintentionally harmed by people who were not developmentally, cognitively, or emotionally appropriate for the interaction. And yet, most of these interactions could have been prevented. There is a growing body of knowledge about animal cognition and emotion that we can draw from to make better educated guesses about how they may experience animal-assisted intervention (AAI) interactions, environments, and activities.

The unconditional love from animals is frequently touted as the foundation for successful AAIs. However, the lines between animal welfare and anthropomorphism are often blurred. For example, if the human handler is enjoying an interaction with a patient in a hospital, it can be difficult for them to objectively view the dog's behavior and assume the dog feels the same way. With concerns of ethics, safety, and liability, AAS welfare must consider both participants (e.g. students, clients, patients) and the animals. We have the responsibility to be stewards to both.

Evolution of Welfare

Over the years, animal welfare has experienced significant evolution. Duncan (2019) describes that until the 17th century, animals had only instrumental value to humans and no rationality. The 1800s

*Corresponding author: Melissa@dogwoodtherapy.com

DOI: 10.1079/9781800622616.0001

brought awareness that animals could suffer, so they gained intrinsic value. Then in the late 20th century, studies included what animals might feel, considering physical and mental well-being based on scientific structure and function, yet focused more on perceptions of stress.

The trail of progressive thinking is clear, but most of the welfare work has been from the utilitarian approach for animals used for agriculture, research, exhibition, and production. Modern academics and practitioners are deviating from the completely utilitarian approach and now contemplating the theory and practice of human–animal interactions and relationships. Animal welfare in the context of AAS is determined by the characteristics of the animal (Glenk, 2017; Enders-Slegers *et al.*, 2019; Ng, 2021) and their perceived experience. AAS are specialty areas that require knowledge and skills in species, breed, and individual traits. In addition, the methods of preparation, communication, training choices, and how these all impact human–animal interactions with students, clients or patients are ultimately the responsibility of the handler.

Improving Animal Welfare with Selection Processes

The selection of a species for AAS should include consideration of the animal's biological make-up. While hedgehogs can be quite social, they are nocturnal, and do best with controlled temperatures. This is not conducive to typical business operating hours and it is difficult to control the conditions of an entire room to match their natural habitat. Turtles may be a good size option, but carry zoonotic risk factors, so handling may not be advisable for vulnerable client populations. Consideration for any species should begin with the investigation of scientifically established species-specific behavioral norms. Due to their popularity, we offer specifics as they pertain to dogs.

Understanding breed-specific traits of dogs can mitigate a lot of frustration. For example, dogs from herding breeds are athletic, energetic, and like to be busy. They are bred to be focused on keeping the herd together which may include heel nipping to navigate another in the right direction and to stay with the group. This may be an unfortunate outcome in pediatrics, but is it fair to try and train this natural genetic predisposition out of them? Is it fair to ask a "ball crazy" dog to work in a nursing facility where all of the residents have tennis balls on the bottom of their walkers? Should we be asking a dog with a fear of loud noises to work in a busy classroom? Handlers must realize that no amount of preparation can guarantee that any animal will necessarily like the job it is being asked to do, but it is less likely if we are asking them to work in an incompatible job.

Impact of Preparation and Training on Welfare

The training techniques used can impact interactions and the outcomes process. For example, a guide, hearing, or service dog is traditionally trained for a one dog *one* person model. This means that a key element, beginning in early training, is that the dog focuses on only one person, the handler. They are trained to avoid social engagement with community-dwelling humans and dogs, to not vocalize, and follow a lot of cues.

A dog being prepared for AAS is trained for a one dog, *many* people model. While the dog will likely have one guardian, it begins training for the social Olympics very early on. He is reinforced and rewarded for approaching and engaging people, for being inquisitive of places and things, and even to politely vocalize in excitement when they see a client approaching. Many clients may have never actually experienced anyone being excited to see them, until they experience AAS.

Preparation for AAS is so much more than obedience training. When clients participate in regular healthcare, education, and human services, the practitioner and client begin to co-regulate. This involves developing a trusting relationship, having structure in the environment, and coaching self-regulation skills (Rosanbalm and Murray, 2017). AAS is another tool that can facilitate the process. How we interact with our animals gives clients information about how we may interact with them. Imagine the client's perception if they observe regular animal interactions as controlling with aversive methods such as choke chains, prong or electrocution collars, or forced participation. Now envision a situation in which we model a trusting relationship, free of physical or emotional punishment, with rich reinforcement and reward-based interactions. We model advocacy skills that are based on the individual dog's preferences, and clients become more confident in advocating for the animal and later, for themselves.

Animals do not share the same complex expressive and receptive communication abilities that humans use, yet they are quite skilled at reading body language. And while they use expressive body language and vocalizations to communicate, the range of human abilities to identify, interpret, and respond to these is broad. Just like humans, animal behavior happens in context and can be subtle. Animals process environmental stimuli such as auditory, olfactory, visual, gustatory, tactile, proprioceptive, vestibular, and interoceptive stimuli differently from humans. Handlers must understand how these impact the experience of the dog. Handlers should also ensure that their dogs get frequent breaks away from people to just enjoy their "dogness" and engage in activities that are enriching to them. For example, dogs sleep 12–15 hours a day and when they are working with us, they should still be able to take frequent naps or take days off from working.

Welfare-guided Team Evaluation

The skills and evaluation of human–dog teams in areas such as therapy and education may look different from that of a team who chooses volunteer visiting. The roles and expectations for each dog vary according to each handler's discipline, range of knowledge and skills, and stylistic approach to their work. There are as many ways to develop a session plan as there are professionals. Different jobs and different skills call for a difference in selection, preparation, and evaluation.

We know that dog behavior and communication occur in context, that is in real time and in direct response to the people, environmental stimuli, and the activities before it. Evaluation should include the handler's ability to predict, recognize, and respond to an animal's communication in the moment. This includes acknowledging that how dogs perceive the behavior of our clients may be different from how our clients intended it. People tend to put unnecessary social pressure on dogs which can cause discomfort. Part of the handler's job is advocating and educating clients about the dog's likes and dislikes, prior to interactions. Just because we can train a dog to do something does not mean that we should ask them to do it. For example, most dogs do not enjoy being patted on the head, being crowded, or being groomed by a clumsy stranger. Is this necessary or can we do better by educating our clients about preferences?

The handler should have skills to set up the dog and client for successful interactions. In addition to preparation and evaluation, it means that our dogs' behaviors and signals should be assessed before, during, and after every session, every time they join us in session. If they are not feeling well, or are uncomfortable with a particular client, we have to pay attention and ameliorate that stressful situation. In addition, considering a dog's aging process, every 52 days is approximately a year to a dog. Just as our preferences and interests change over time, so do those of our dogs, just at a much faster rate. We recommend that objective evaluations occur, by a skilled veterinarian or dog trainer with behavior experience, in context—including the population, environment, and representation of activity skill sets—at least yearly. Good welfare also includes regular health checks by a qualified veterinarian.

Welfare does not stop with preparation of the handler and dog. We must ensure that each potential client is screened for participation in AAS. Some considerations include assessing developmental levels. Young children and others with cognitive disabilities may not have the skills to follow directions, lack impulse control, or may mouth/eat things off the floor—including toys that dogs have mouthed. These behaviors increase zoonotic risk factors and make for an unsafe situation for the dog.

Understanding the client's history and perception of animals is critical to avoid further trauma to the client or the dog. People with physical disabilities may not be able to control the pressure or location of a friendly stroke of a dog's fur. They may lose balance bending over to greet a dog, or unintentionally move their wheelchair when the dog's tail is under the wheel. Handlers should be able to predict and help prevent anything that could possibly go wrong.

Conclusion and Recommendations

AASs are a worthwhile pursuit; however, specialty training for both handler and dog is required. This may include formal university certificate programs or continuing education programs or coursework. Any of these options should include a hands-on component. Membership of professional

---

organizations can also be used to provide practitioners with standards, competencies, and ongoing continuing education.

Bibliography

Animal Assisted Intervention International (2020) *Animal Assisted Intervention*. Available at: https://aai-int. org/aai/animal-assisted-intervention/ (accessed 15 March 2023).

Duncan, I.J.H. (2019) Animal welfare: a brief history. In: Hild, S. and Schweitzer, L. (eds) *Animal Welfare: From Science to Law*. Conference proceedings by La Fondation Droit Animal, Éthique et Sciences, pp. 13–20. Available at: https://www.fondation-droit -animal.org/documents/AnimalWelfare2019.v1.pdf (accessed 15 March 2023).

Elischer, M. (2019) The five freedoms: a history lesson in animal care and welfare. Michigan State University. Available at: https://www.canr.msu.edu/news/an_ animal_welfare_history_lesson_on_the_five_freedoms #:~:text=In%20summary%2C%20the%20report %20stated,detail%20list%20of%20the%20needs (accessed 15 March 2023).

Enders-Slegers, M., Hediger, K., Beetz, A., Jegatheesan, B. and Turner, D. (2019) Animal-assisted interventions within an international perspective: trends, research, and practices. In: Fine, A.H. (ed.) *Handbook on Animal-Assisted Therapy: Foundations and Guidelines for Animal-Assisted Interventions*, 5th edn. Academic Press, Cambridge, Massachusetts, pp. 464–477.

Glenk, L.M. (2017) Current perspectives on therapy dog welfare in animal-Assisted interventions. *Animals* 7(2), 7. DOI: 10.3390/ani7020007.

Jegatheesan, B. (2018) IAHAIO White Paper 2014, updated for 2018. International Association of Human-Animal Interaction Organizations (IAHAIO). Available at: https://iahaio.org/wp/wp-content/uploads/2021/01/ iahaio-white-paper-2018-english.pdf (accessed 13 July 2023).

Mellor, D.J. (2016) Updating animal welfare thinking: moving beyond the "five freedoms" towards "a life worth living". *Animals* 6(3), 21. DOI: 10.3390/ ani6030021.

Mellor, D.J. (2017) Operational details of the five domains model and its key applications to the assessment and management of animal welfare. *Animals* 7(8), 60. DOI: 10.3390/ani7080060.

Michaels, L. (2017) *Do No Harm: Dog Training and Behavior Manual*. Self-published, San Diego, California.

Ng, Z. (2021) Strategies to assessing and enhancing animal welfare in animal-assisted interventions. In: Peralta, J.M. and Fine, A.F. (eds) *The Welfare of Animals in Animal-Assisted Interventions*. Springer, Cham, Switzerland, pp. 123–154. DOI: 10.1007/978-3-030-69587-3.

Rosanbalm, K.D. and Murray, D.W. (2017) *Caregiver Co-Regulation Across Development: A Practice Brief OPRE Brief #2017-80*. Office of Planning, Research, and Evaluation (OPRE), Administration for Children and Families, US Department of Health and Human Services, Washington, DC.

2 Standards of Practice and Professional Competencies to Protect Welfare and Promote Thriving in AAI

Taylor Chastain Griffin*

Pet Partners, Association of Animal-Assisted Intervention Professionals (AAAIP), Bellevue, Washington, USA

Abstract

It was concern for therapy animal welfare that originally motivated the author to seek as much education and opportunity as possible within the field of animal-assisted interventions (AAIs). With a background as a dog trainer, her first true career aspiration was to implement her own therapy animals into her mental health counseling practice. However, upon just getting started in her fieldwork internship, she noted how few resources existed for professionals who want to incorporate the power of the human–animal bond into their work. She also noted how many professionals with impressive expertise relating to their human services vocation lacked information specific to animal behavior, making it impossible to serve as competent advocates for the welfare and well-being of their animal counterparts. This discovery led her to positions of leadership at Pet Partners and the Association of Animal-Assisted Intervention Professionals—two organizations whose central focus revolves around protecting the welfare of all involved in AAIs.

Key Terminology

According to the American Veterinary Medical Association, animal welfare can be conceptualized as how an animal is coping through lived experiences over time (AVMA, 2022). What are the common states that an animal experiences? Is the environment comfortable and safe with the provision of appropriate nutrition and exercise (mentally and physically)? Is the animal able to freely express preferences and natural behaviors? The protection of an animal's welfare is not only core to securing a high quality of life, but it is absolutely essential for the safety and well-being of all who are involved in animal-assisted interventions (AAIs). As so powerfully stated by author and trainer Pelar (2023), "behavior deteriorates under stress". If the welfare of therapy animals is not upheld, the intervention becomes less effective, higher in risk, and unethical for both the animal and the client.

The field of AAI is filled with many different terms and associated acronyms which can be further explored in Fig. 2.1. AAI is an umbrella term that encompasses the different kinds of activities that therapy animals are involved in and is built upon the principle of the human–animal bond. The protection of animal welfare across all therapy animal activities promotes this bond in a way that facilitates the positive impacts of AAI.

The importance of welfare for therapy animals is captured in the very definition of the term. Therapy animals are those that have been evaluated on their ability to safely interact with a wide range of populations—together with their handlers who are trained in best practices to ensure

---

*Taylorc@petpartners.org

© CAB International 2024. *Animal-assisted Interventions: Recognizing and Mitigating Potential Welfare Challenges* (ed. L.R. Kogan)
DOI: 10.1079/9781800622616.0002

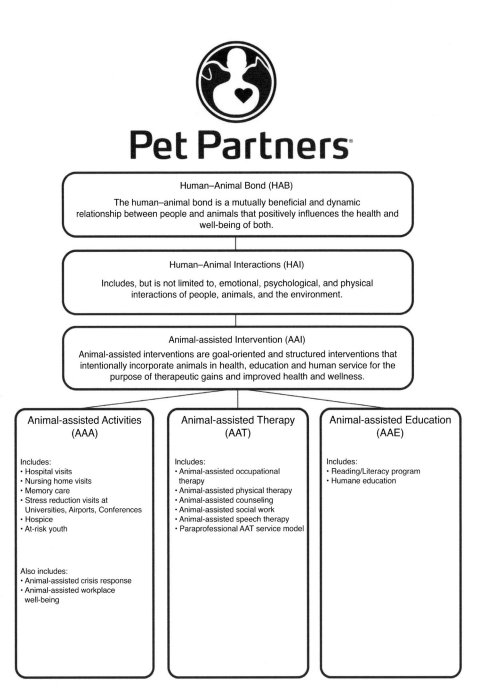

Fig. 2.1. Pet Partners' animal-assisted interventions (AAIs) terminology.

effective interactions that support animal welfare. Therapy animals don't simply tolerate their role. They should exhibit behaviors that indicate active enjoyment. Regardless of the species, therapy animals should be highly affiliative in nature, meaning that they freely initiate interactions with people outside of those they know. They should not be overly taxed by travel, and they should be able to quickly recover from any new stimuli they might experience as stressful. They should have a developed relationship with their handler that allows the pair to clearly communicate with one another while empowering the handler to advocate for their needs.

Protective AAI Resources

There are many resources that go beyond the simple protection of animal welfare within AAI by promoting a sense of thriving for the animals involved in this work. First is the Standards of Practice in Animal-Assisted Interventions (available at: https://therapyanimalstandards.org/ (accessed February 20 2023)). This document includes five sections that address standards for handlers, therapy animals, assessment, animal welfare, and risk management. Additionally, there are two sections that offer recommendations for facilities seeking to incorporate therapy animals and for researchers pursuing AAI topics. This document includes foundational considerations including:

- The role of the therapy animal handler and the knowledge, skills, and aptitude they should possess to ensure effective and safe interactions.
- Temperament, health, and training standards for therapy animals, along with best practices in assessing an animal's suitability for AAI.
- The articulation and concrete examples of welfare in action including an animal's demonstration of active consent, AAI time limitations, and the use of non-coercive equipment.

In addition to the standards that are in place for therapy animal programming in general, there are competencies and best practices specific to professionals who work with therapy animals as a part of their vocational practice. The Association of Animal-Assisted Intervention Professionals (AAAIP) is a sister organization to Pet Partners, created in 2022, to better serve the needs of those who implement therapy animals into formal treatment or educational plans. By working with subject matter experts and undergoing various processes of empirical validation, AAAIP's published competencies include the attitudes, knowledge, skills, and abilities required of professional AAI practitioners. These competencies include a code of ethics to provide a set of wide-ranging, non-specific principles that govern decision making in AAI. Subsequently, this publicly available field resource (available at: https://www.aaaiponline. org/resources (accessed March 1 2023)) includes a code of conduct that provides specific practices and behavior recommendations for those practicing AAI. Throughout each of these guiding documents, the intention remains the same: to protect the welfare of both the people and the animals involved in AAI.

Practical Strategies to Protect Therapy Animal Welfare

In addition to becoming aware of the supportive resources that are available to guide therapy animal handlers on the humane and ethical application of AAI, it can be extremely helpful to learn from the experiences of other AAI professionals who have had to work through welfare considerations in applied settings. Having assisted in the training process of hundreds of dogs (and even a handful of cats and pigs!) and having partnered with many therapy animals of my own, it is my hope that the applied best practices I've learned along the way are beneficial to others who are getting started in this space.

1. Learn to communicate with your animal

This is a sentiment that seems obvious on the surface but is actually deeply personal, complex, and unique to each human–animal duo. The more animals I've shared my life with, the more I realize the power of developing a communication system that is tailored to each animal's skills and interests. At the core, I believe in establishing a solid working relationship with our animals through a training relationship that relies on positive training methodologies. I use a mix of verbal and physical cues to establish a language with my animals while also being mindful not to ask my animals to perform outside of their preferences. Though it is essential that any therapy animal handler learns general body language principles of the species that they partner with, a handler must also take time to notice the way that their animal uniquely expresses themselves. For example, my retired therapy dog Lucy (a Yorkipoo) often trembles slightly with excitement upon first entering a new facility. For many dogs, trembling is a sign of negative stress, but for

Lucy, given that this is accompanied with other body language cues such as approaching behaviors, play bowing, and initiating petting, is indicative of a positive state brought about by an initial burst of stimuli.

2. Practice consent testing

In every single interaction in which a therapy animal is involved, they should have the ability to freely express the desire to take space from the client. Petting consent tests are a great way to determine how an animal is experiencing a new interaction. This entails allowing a person to pet the animal briefly, and then stop and watch the animal for approaching or retreating behaviors. This is a test that is not only helpful in protecting therapy animal well-being but can also be a powerful tool to model boundary setting and safe touching for professionals who focus on those subjects within their existing treatment plans.

3. Prioritize your animal's preferences

The role of a therapy animal looks different for all animals involved in the interactions. The environment, population, and treatment planning/activity structuring involved in AAI should reflect the therapy animal at the individual level. While some of my dogs thrive in loud, populated settings, other dogs prefer quieter, one-on-one environments. Some of my dogs demonstrate an affinity for working with very young populations while others excel working with people at the end of their life. Rex, my retired border collie, loves few things more than a game of fetch. With that in mind, fetching was often incorporated into my treatment planning with clients. If we set our animals up to enjoy their role and reward them according to their preferences, we take a significant step in encouraging them to thrive in AAI.

4. Thoughtful preparation of the AAI environment

Along with selecting an environment that is the best fit for your animal, there are essential steps to take to prepare that setting in a way that enhances your animal's comfort. Therapy animals should have a safe, comfortable place to retreat to at any time they wish to do so. They should have access to clean water, frequent bio breaks, and should be continuously monitored for signs of stress or exhaustion. While therapy animals partnering with volunteers in animal-assisted activities (AAA) are held to a 2-hour time limit on visits, AAI professionals might work with therapy animals for longer work days. Regardless of the specifics surrounding the animal's time limit, the handler should be prepared to end sessions as needed based on the animal's body language.

5. All parties play a role in welfare

Though a therapy animal's handler is ultimately responsible for safeguarding the well-being of their animal, it's my belief that all people involved in the intervention can play a role as an advocate for the animal. When approaching new people or preparing clients, handlers are encouraged to find age-appropriate ways to communicate the importance of making sure the animal is comfortable. For example, handlers should instruct clients how best to pet the animal. Additionally, prior to a client interacting with an animal, they should be informed that, based on the animal's needs and body language, the session might need to end unexpectedly. In mental health counseling settings, I would often preemptively educate my clients on the body language cues we would be looking for to assess stress in my therapy dogs. Few moments were more rewarding than when a client would notice a sign of slight stress, even before I did, and would suggest an adjustment to make the animal more comfortable.

6. Practice outside of sessions

The AAI experience is often a novel situation for both the animal and the handler. Whenever possible, expose your animal to new stimuli outside of AAI sessions. Go to places like animal-friendly retail stores together to watch your animal's body language, practice directing people through interactions with your pet, and further develop your means of communicating with your animal in real-life settings.

7. Maintain humility as a lifelong learner

Involvement with AAI is a journey, an exciting, fulfilling one that has no final, fixed destination. Therapy animal handlers should assume the position of lifelong learners who stay actively engaged in emerging research, education, and professional communities to stay up to date on the latest best practices related to therapy animal welfare.

I believe in the profound power of the human–animal bond, and it is the sincere goal of my career to make therapy animal programming more accessible to as many people as possible. However, with the commitment to bring therapy animals to wider populations, there must also be a commitment to standardized practices that protect the welfare of the animals who so meaningfully share their love with us.

References

American Veterinary Medical Association (AVMA) (2022) Animal welfare: what is it? AVMA. Available at: https://www.avma.org/resources/animal-health-welfare/animal-welfare-what-it (accessed 30 March 2023).

Pelar, C. (2023) Living with kids and dogs. Colleen Pelar, 21 February. Available at: https://colleenpelar.com/livingwithkidsanddogs/ (accessed 30 March 2023).

3 Welfare and Well-being Considerations in Dog Selection and Involvement in Animal-assisted Interventions

Risë VanFleet*

International Institute for Animal Assisted Play Therapy®, Boiling Springs, Pennsylvania, USA

Abstract

This chapter explores the competencies of animal-assisted intervention (AAI) handlers, including the selection of dogs for AAI work. The importance of mutually respectful and responsive relationships with dogs within the realm of AAI is emphasized. It is critically important that throughout the life of the human–dog partnership, handlers ensure the well-being of *both* humans and animals, based upon the species-specific and individual needs of the dogs *and* those of the clients.

Introduction

It is far too common for websites depicting animal-assisted interventions (AAIs) to show images of dogs displaying behavioral signs of disinterest, discomfort, and stress. These images are often accompanied by positive commentary about the wonderful benefits of AAI for its human participants. While the benefits of animals for people in therapeutic settings are well documented (e.g. Friedmann and Son, 2009; Chandler, 2017; Tedeschi and Jenkins, 2019), the animals' experiences have been, until recently, largely ignored. Yet, it is important to consider their experiences in AAI to ensure that our animal partners are not only comfortable, but actually enjoy themselves.

Today, few would argue that dogs are sentient beings with emotions, preferences, and cognitive processes. It behooves practitioners to treat them as such, and this has implications for how one selects and works with animals in their daily lives as well as in AAIs (Peralta, 2021). The growing body of research on dogs' well-being needs greater attention in the AAI community (McGreevy *et al.*, 2012; Mellor *et al.*, 2020; Cobb *et al.*, 2021; MacLean *et al.*, 2021; Peralta and Fine, 2021; Giraudet *et al.*, 2022). It is critical that handlers ensure the well-being of *both* humans and animals based on the species-specific and individual needs of the dogs *and* the clients.

Therapist/Handler Competencies for AAI

Before an animal is involved in AAI, it is important that the therapist or handler (henceforth, handler) begins their own competency development needed for this work. These competencies include the skills to conduct the actual interventions, such as therapy or teaching skills, but also extend considerably beyond one's human interaction skills. To include animals as partners means one must learn a great deal about the involved species, the breed or mix of breeds, and especially the individual animal.

The extensive competencies required have been outlined in some detail (VanFleet, 2014, 2018,

---

*Rise@risevanfleet.com

© CAB International 2024. *Animal-assisted Interventions: Recognizing and Mitigating Potential Welfare Challenges* (ed. L.R. Kogan)
DOI: 10.1079/9781800622616.0003

2022a; Stewart *et al.*, 2016; VanFleet and Faa-Thompson, 2017; Johnson *et al.*, 2020; Kerulo *et al.*, 2020). In addition to the human skills, they include animal-related knowledge and skills, such as: (i) observation skills; (ii) detailed working knowledge of dogs' body language (Rugaas, 2006; Byrnes, 2008); (iii) knowledge of the ethology and natural behavior of dogs (McConnell, 2002); (iv) handling skills; (v) positive training skills; and (vi) knowledge and advocacy for the dog's welfare and well-being (Mellor *et al.*, 2020). They also include the ability to split one's attention between client and dog, and to anticipate potential stressful conditions through the use of proactive attention. Additionally, competencies are required in building and maintaining healthy relationships with one's dogs including the ability to engage in reciprocal relationships that honor the dogs' preferences, choices, and agency, and facilitation skills that consider the dog as much as the client when interventions are applied (VanFleet, 2020).

All of this is a far cry from the popular, but risky, practice of "taking one's nice family dog to work". There are many important considerations of the dog's needs that must be considered before incorporating the dog into clinical, educational, or support work.

Building a Relationship and Preparing Dogs for Participation in AAI

Not all dogs are suitable for therapy work. In general, dogs who are friendly, interested in people, curious, attentive, confident, and without significant behavior problems have the potential for AAIs. A qualified canine professional can assist with the selection of puppies or dogs with the right features, but there is no guarantee that a new dog will be suitable. Whether one acquires a puppy or adopts a dog, a period of time is needed to get to know the unique dog and build a reciprocal and secure relationship. Not only must the puppy or dog adjust to the new home environment, but positive socialization experiences are needed so they become comfortable with many different people, places, and objects.

The best type of relationship between dog and handler for therapy work is a reciprocal partnership (VanFleet and Faa-Thompson, 2017). It is based on collaboration rather than a controlling,

obedience-oriented approach (VanFleet and Faa-Thompson, 2011a, 2011b). While dogs do need to learn how to behave politely in the human world, the handler should give them voice and choice whenever possible, and then listen and try to accommodate the dogs' needs for exploration, play, connection, decision making, exercise, and rest. Training should use positive, dog-friendly methods and therapists should respect the dogs as individuals and avoid any depersonalizing interactions. Most of all, they should enjoy each other's company. As with human relationships, this type of mutually beneficial relationship between human and dog takes time. This type of relationship is indispensable in AAIs and provides a model and metaphor of healthy relationships for clients and students.

Most AAI practitioners want to have good relationships with their animals and often believe they have this. Even so, there are always improvements that can be made in awareness, empathy, and adaptation to the dog's needs. Only when practitioners develop the aforementioned competencies through considerable training and supervision do they realize what an enormous task it is to conduct AAIs with full attention to the dogs' needs. At the same time, developing these types of reciprocal relationships leads to enormously satisfying lives together at work and home.

Evaluating and Selecting Dogs for AAIs

Most AAI programs require dogs to be at least 1–2 years old and developmentally mature enough to be assessed for therapy work. Many AAI programs evaluate dogs' behavioral reactions upon being exposed to situations they might face in a hospital or school. Some assessments expose dogs to increasing levels of stress to determine at which point the dog displays stress signals. Most of these tests have been developed for traditional AAI environments, but there are some shortcomings if applying this selection method across the board. Different types of environments and therapeutic or educational "jobs" might require different characteristics. While one would want a calm, quiet dog for a hospital environment, a more active, playful dog might work best in an outdoor program or in Animal Assisted Play Therapy™ (AAPT).

An alternative method for selecting dogs for therapy work uses the "goodness of fit" model drawn from child development. In the goodness-of-fit approach, a non-stressful and often play-based assessment is made of the dog's personality, including their preferences and typical choices, on multiple dimensions. In the Animal Appropriateness Scale (VanFleet, in press), for example, each of four dimensions—physiological/sensory functioning, social functioning, adaptability, and psychological functioning—contain six to eight characteristics to be observed and coded. Items such as energy level, interest and engagement, ability to focus, self-regulation, independence, sociability, and patience are operationalized and scored by both the handler and someone trained to make such observations in multiple settings. At no time are the dogs stressed to ascertain their responses, instead, play-based methods of "asking" the dog's preferences and interests are used. The Clothier Animal Response Assessment Tool (CARAT) (Clothier, 2023) is another useful tool that can be used for the purpose of identifying personality features.

After a profile is created, the appropriate type of AAI is built around the dog's needs and personality (VanFleet, 2022b). This method has been used in AAPT where the therapist develops interventions based simultaneously on: (i) client goals; (ii) the dog's personality, abilities, and preferences; (iii) the therapist's orientation and skills; and (iv) the environment within which they work. In this way, a more animal-friendly approach is provided by adapting to what the dog might enjoy. Handlers also develop a Therapy Involvement Plan (TIP) for each animal based on this profile. The TIP defines the individual dog's natural behaviors and preferences and then identifies the best "job". This process requires handlers to see their dogs clearly for who they are and to include them only in AAIs that are a good fit.

What Does This Mean for Actual Practice of AAI?

For the sake of the dogs, as well as the clients, it is essential that handlers develop and use these competencies at all times. This type of empathic and reciprocal relationship provides greater attention to the welfare needs of the dogs, as defined by the dogs themselves, and creates a far more satisfying partnership. It also offers a metaphor for the therapeutic relationship with clients who have much to gain from seeing models of mutually beneficial relationships.

References

Byrnes, C. (2008) *What Is My Dog Saying? Canine Communication 101*. [CD-ROM]. Diamonds in the Ruff, Spokane, Washington State.

Chandler, C.K. (2017) *Animal-Assisted Therapy in Counseling*, 3rd edn. Routledge, New York. DOI: 10.4324/9781315673042.

Clothier, S. (2023) CARAT the Clothier Animal Response Assessment Tool. Available at: https://suzanneclothier.com/carat/ (accessed 2 March 2023).

Cobb, M.L., Otto, C.M. and Fine, A.H. (2021) The animal welfare science of working dogs: current perspectives on recent advances and future directions. *Frontiers in Veterinary Science* 8, 666898. DOI: 10.3389/fvets.2021.666898.

Friedmann, E. and Son, H. (2009) The human-companion animal bond: how humans benefit. *The Veterinary Clinics of North America: Small Animal Practice* 39(2), 293–326. DOI: 10.1016/j.cvsm.2008.10.015.

Giraudet, C.S.E., Liu, K., McElligott, A.G. and Cobb, M. (2022) Are children and dogs best friends? A scoping review to explore the positive and negative effects of child-dog interactions. *PeerJ* 10, e14532. DOI: 10.7717/peerj.14532.

Johnson, A., VanFleet, R., Stewart, L., Crowley, S., De Prekel, M. *et al.* (2020) Summary of considerations for APA ethical standards: competencies in animal-assisted interventions. Position statement for APA Division 17, Section 13. Available at: https://www.human-animal-interaction.org/ (accessed 14 March 2023).

Kerulo, G., Kargas, N., Mills, D.S., Law, G., VanFleet, R. *et al.* (2020) Animal-assisted interventions: relationship between standards and qualifications. *People and Animals: The International Journal of Research and Practice* 3(1), Article4. Available at: https://docs.lib.purdue.edu/paij/vol3/iss1/4 (accessed 2 March 2023).

MacLean, E.L., Fine, A., Herzog, H., Strauss, E. and Cobb, M.L. (2021) The new era of canine science: reshaping our relationships with dogs. *Frontiers in Veterinary Science* 8, 675782. DOI: 10.3389/fvets.2021.675782.

McConnell, P.B. (2002) *The Other End of the Leash: Why We Do What We Do Around Dogs*. Ballantine Books, New York.

McGreevy, P.D., Starling, M., Branson, N.J., Cobb, M.L. and Calnon, D. (2012) An overview of the dog–human dyad and ethograms within it. *Journal of Veterinary Behavior* 7(2), 103–117. DOI: 10.1016/j.jveb.2011.06.001.

Mellor, D.J., Beausoleil, N.J., Littlewood, K.E., McLean, A.N., McGreevy, P.D. *et al.* (2020) The 2020 five domains model: including human-animal interactions in assessments of animal welfare. *Animals* 10(10), 1870. DOI: 10.3390/ani10101870.

Peralta, J.M. (2021) The animals' perspective and its impact on welfare during animal-assisted interventions. In: Peralta, J.M. and Fine, A.F. (eds) *The Welfare of Animals in Animal-Assisted Interventions*. Springer, Cham, Switzerland, pp. 1–20. DOI: 10.1007/978-3-030-69587-3.

Peralta, J.M. and Fine, A.H. (eds) (2021) *The Welfare of Animals in Animal-Assisted Interventions*. Springer, Cham, Switzerland. DOI: 10.1007/978-3-030-69587-3.

Rugaas, T. (2006) *On Talking Terms with Dogs: Calming Signals*, 2nd edn. Dogwise Publishing, Wenatchee, Washington State.

Stewart, L.A., Chang, C.Y., Parker, L.K. and Grubbs, N. (2016) *Animal-Assisted Therapy in Counselling Competencies*. American Counselling Association, Mental Health Interest Network, Alexandria, Virginia. Available at: https://www.counseling.org/docs/default-source/competencies/animal-assisted-therapy-competencies-june-2016.pdf (accessed 2 March 2023).

Tedeschi, P. and Jenkins, M.A. (eds) (2019) *Transforming Trauma: Resilience and Healing Through our Connections with Animals*. Purdue University Press, West Lafayette, Indiana. DOI: 10.2307/j.ctv2x00vgg.

VanFleet, R. (2014) What it means to be humane in animal-assisted interventions. *The APDT Chronicle of the Dog Fall* 18–20. Available at: https://risevanfleet.com/wp-content/uploads/2023/01/HUMANE.in_.AAI_.article-RV.pdf (accessed 2 March 2023).

VanFleet, R. (2018) What type of training do therapy dogs need? International Institute for Animal Assisted Play Therapy®, Boiling Springs, Pennsylvania. Available at: https://iiaapt.org/training/ (accessed 3 March 2023).

VanFleet, R. (2020) Do we sell them short? Supporting "agency" in animals. International Institute for Animal Assisted Play Therapy, Boiling Springs, Pennsylvania. Available at: https://iiaapt.org/do-we-sell-them-short-supporting-agency-in-animals/ (accessed 2 March 2023).

VanFleet, R. (2022a) Why competencies for professionals in animal assisted interventions? International Institute for Animal Assisted Play Therapy, Boiling Springs, Pennsylvania. Available at: https://iiaapt.org/why-competencies-for-professionals-in-animal-assisted-interventions/ (accessed 2 March 2023).

VanFleet, R. (2022b) Professional decision-making in Animal Assisted Play Therapy™: how the goodness-of-fit model impacts practice. Available at: https://iiaapt.org/professional-decision-making-in-animal-assisted-play-therapy-how-the-goodness-of-fit-model-impacts-practice/ (accessed 2 March 2023).

VanFleet, R. (in press) The Animal Appropriateness Scale™: a tool for assessing key characteristics of potential therapy animals. International Institute for Animal Assisted Play Therapy®, Boiling Springs, Pennsylvania.

VanFleet, R. and Faa-Thompson, T. (2011a) Control, compassion, and choices (part 1). *The APDT Chronicle of the Dog* July/August 50–53. Available at: https://iiaapt.org/control-compassion-and-choices-part-i/ (accessed 2 March 2023).

VanFleet, R. and Faa-Thompson, T. (2011b) Control, compassion, and choices (part 2). *The APDT Chronicle of the Dog* September/October 28–33. Available at: https://iiaapt.org/control-compassion-and-choices-part-2/ (accessed 2 March 2023).

VanFleet, R. and Faa-Thompson, T. (2017) *Animal Assisted Play Therapy*. Professional Resource Press, Sarasota, Florida.

4 Equine Welfare in Therapy and Learning Services: an Overview

Nina Ekholm Fry*

Institute for Human-Animal Connection, University of Denver, Denver, Colorado, USA

Abstract

The importance of the welfare and well-being of horses that are part of human health and learning services is receiving ongoing attention through research studies, scientific summaries, and practice guidelines. This chapter addresses these issues by first providing a brief overview of horses involved in human services, followed by a discussion of practitioner attitudes pertaining to horses, and the needs of horses in terms of their living environment and handling practices. Finally, there is an explanation of five key areas of responsibility for practitioners during human–horse interactions proposed by the author with the intention of improving horse welfare.

Introduction

Thoughtful people who are involved in animal-assisted interventions recognize that human welfare matters, animal welfare matters, and the two are closely connected.

(Fraser, 2021, p. viii)

The importance of the welfare and well-being of horses who are part of human health and learning services is receiving ongoing attention through research studies (e.g. Merkies *et al.*, 2018), scientific summaries (e.g. Ekholm Fry, 2021), and practice guidelines (e.g. IAHAIO, 2021). It may feel particularly salient to focus on the well-being of horses when they are part of human healthcare and learning services as human care ethics are already involved in the service delivery. However, the context of human services does not automatically offer protection against the lack of recognition and mitigation of equine welfare issues. It is up to each person involved to allow new learning and welfare-enhancing practices to become part of the everyday handling of the horses we care so much about.

Horses in Human Services and Adjacent Areas: a Brief Overview

When referring to horses in human services, it can be useful to recognize that there are different human service and activity areas where horses are involved. There are common welfare issues across these areas, which I will discuss briefly in this introductory chapter, and also issues specific to the service or activity provided as the tasks the horse is expected to perform vary.

When referring to treatment or therapy that includes interactions with horses or the movement of the horse, the human profession defines the service, not the fact that a horse is present. Examples include physical therapy, occupational therapy, and speech therapy where equine movement is used as a treatment tool as part of the larger treatment plan. Similarly, equine interactions can be incorporated into the process of psychotherapy and clinical mental health counseling as a therapy technique within the therapy approaches the

*Nina.ekholm-fry@du.edu

DOI: 10.1079/9781800622616.0004

licensed therapist employs. Horses can also be part of learning services that are based on educational constructs and focused on goals related to, for instance, life skills or academic achievement. Adjacent areas that do not constitute a human service but may be relevant in this context are adaptive/therapeutic riding and volunteer visits to hospitals and schools. Adaptive riding and horsemanship lessons, also known as therapeutic riding, provides access to horses and riding activities for those who experience physical, cognitive, or mental health-related barriers for recreating with horses in typical equestrian settings without accommodations. Visits to hospitals and schools are typically conducted by a volunteer with the purpose of providing a pleasant social encounter. In the USA, a miniature horse can function as a service animal but welfare concerns for this role falls outside the scope of this discussion.

Practitioner Attitudes and "Horse Culture"

How we think, talk, and act around horses, which defines our personal *horse culture*, greatly affect whether we regularly encounter new, science-based information about horses, and if so, what we do with it. There are many reasons why a person may not actively mitigate equine welfare issues: (i) they may not perceive that there is a problem; (ii) they may misinterpret communication from the horse; (iii) they may follow incorrect advice from someone who they believe is an expert; or (iv) they may be exposed to situations that create compromised equine welfare so often that the issues are not recognized due to being common occurrences. In addition, I would argue that there exists a so-called toughness culture in the horse world for both people and horses due to the size of the horse and the working conditions in the horse industry overall. There seems to be an expectation of high physical impact, such as an occurrence of biting and striking from horses, and an overall expectation to "suck it up" for both people and horses. This may negatively influence the pursuit of recognizing nuanced communication from horses and changing existing management practices that have welfare consequences when horses are part of human services. Care is not welfare—our well-meaning care for horses does not necessarily correlate with good welfare for them.

It can be a bit awkward to realize that we as humans have inherent cognitive barriers to considering the perspective of horses in our interactions with them, despite our best intentions. One of these cognitive tendencies is thinking primarily about human benefits and values. An example is, "this is so good for humans so it can't be bad for horses—they enjoy it too". Another cognitive tendency is to emphasize how different the horse is from us, using labels such as "prey animal" and "unpredictable", while making statements that imply that the horse understands human-specific concepts such as healthcare ("the horse is a therapist and I let them take care of themselves"). These examples create situations where the horse's vulnerable position is underestimated and sufficient action is not being taken to change the circumstances that lead to reduced welfare, whether the horse is standing in cross-ties with little option to move away, being led by someone who is not paying attention to lead-rope pressure, or being sat on without appropriately fitted equipment that distributes weight across their back.

Asking ourselves the question, "Just because we can, does it mean we should?" is a good start for exploring our equine interactions in a systematic way and questioning long-standing traditions. Otherwise, we may inadvertently hinder ourselves from recognizing an issue and seeking out new information about it. In many instances, science-based guidance for how to improve welfare of horses within our human pursuits is available but because it does not fully fit with what we already know, we come up with reasons to reject it.

Living Environment and Handling Practices

Much is known about the needs of horses in their living environment in general and the potential for positive and negative impacts from our direct handling of them. Still, management practices that go directly against the needs of horses despite knowledge of other options are prevalent in the horse industry overall. The most basic needs of horses include free movement, forage, social housing, and choice in their everyday life. These examples arise from scientific study of equine behavior and health. For instance, we may be able to calculate the exact calories a horse needs on a given day but we must also understand the equine welfare needs for feeding behaviors, which include near-constant access to fiber in the form of hay or grass to facilitate time spent chewing, a low head position, and slow movement while eating.

Attitudes such as, "horses need to come in at night" to a small box stall and run (horses will, of course, appear to eagerly want to go into their stalls if this is the place they are fed grain), practices such as blanketing horses with unaltered coats at 40°F (4.4°C), or only providing small portions of hay at "breakfast, lunch, and dinner" if no other fiber is available, all constitute considerable equine welfare violations and we need to be honest about that. Some providers may feel that benefits for participants in human services are so great that they are willing to overlook mental or physical discomfort in the horse, even if they recognize it. An example of this is to continuously include a horse in human services who regularly nips or threatens to bite during interactions. When I am told about this, which I consider a serious welfare issue for all involved, the most common explanation provided is that it is a problem with a particular horse and not related to possible welfare deficits in how horses are made to live their lives each day, also outside of the direct human interaction.

There has been some research interest in whether the human's emotional state has welfare consequences for the horse in therapy or learning sessions (see e.g. Merkies *et al.*, 2018). It is likely that horses, similar to humans, have different tolerance thresholds for tension and other states in humans due to a variety of factors, including their prior experiences with humans and aspects of their personality and temperament. Skilled selection of horses comfortable with interactions is therefore particularly important. In addition, experiences of human emotionality as part of therapy or education services does not seem to be *more* significant than what the human does to the horse during the interaction. This requires us to pay particular attention to how horses are handled by participants and carefully assess practices that we may assume are preferred by horses, such as grooming (Schroeder *et al.*, 2023). Practitioners who include horses in human therapy and learning services should base their handling and training practices on the physical, mental, and sensory capacities of horses, and on the science of how horses learn and communicate. This includes attention to the individual horse's

sensory load and a focus on reinforcement in training protocols.

Finally, conversations about agency and choice for horses in their interactions with humans are becoming more prevalent. It may be valuable to look to concepts like the Lundy (2007) model of participation (space, voice, audience, and influence) and the Substance Abuse and Mental Health Services Administration (SAMHSA) principles of a trauma-informed approach for guidance in our interactions with horses as we hold structural power over them.

Practitioner Responsibilities During Human–Horse Interactions

I have previously proposed five areas of responsibilities that a practitioner providing a therapy or learning service has during direct interactions between a service participant and the horse with the intention of positively impacting welfare (Ekholm Fry, 2021). They are summarized below.

1. Monitor interactions and track affective states

When a participant is interacting with the horse, you must watch the interaction at all times so that you can track the emotional states of both the horse and the person without interruption.

2. Assess and address handling and touch

When a participant is touching the horse or otherwise handling their body or using equipment like a lead rope, you must assess the interaction continuously and address anything that exceeds minimal pressure without delay.

3. Communicate accurately about the horse and the interaction

When you are describing ways to have relationally appropriate interactions with the horses or even the horse's role in the service you are providing, it is imperative that you do not mislead the client with scientifically incorrect statements such as, "the horse mirrors your feelings".

4. Assess stress

When you are planning for or monitoring interactions, you must watch for levels of undue stress in the horse, noting their individual preferences and capacities, and modify without delay.

5. Promote positive states

As much as possible during any given interaction or session, you should strive to promote positive states in the horses, such as relaxation, and providing them with hay if they are expected to stand still for prolonged periods of time.

Conclusions

I have no doubt that you, the reader, are one of those thoughtful people David Fraser refers to in the opening quote of this chapter, and that you want to prevent harmful situations when including horses in therapy and education services. However, the time has come to understand the difference between our good intentions and the impact of our actions. This includes asking ourselves whether it is reasonable to have horses part of human services who are not able to move freely during the day or night, who are fasting for longer than 3–4 hours at a time, and who are not housed together with other horses due to lack of space. It takes courage to advocate for and to make change against the backdrop of a horse industry that is not always treating horses well. Change is hard, cultural shifts even harder, but it is the direction we must take toward a more just future for horses and people alike.

References

Ekholm Fry, N. (2021) Welfare considerations for horses in therapy and education services. In: Peralta, J.M. and Fine, A.H. (eds) *The Welfare of Animals in Animal-Assisted Interventions*. Springer, Cham, Switzerland, pp. 219–242. DOI: 10.1007/978-3-030-69587-3.

Fraser, D. (2021) Foreword. In: Peralta, J.M. and Fine, A.H. (eds) *The Welfare of Animals in Animal-Assisted Interventions*. Springer, Cham, Switzerland, pp. vii–ix.

International Association of Human–Animal Interaction Organizations (IAHAIO) (2021) IAHAIO international guidelines on care, training and welfare requirements for equines in equine-assisted services. Available at: https://iahaio.org/iahaio-international-guidelines-on-care-training-and-welfare-requirements-for-equines-in-equine-assisted-services/ (accessed 18 March 2023).

Lundy, L. (2007) Voice is not enough: conceptualising article 12 of the United Nations Convention on the rights of the child. *British Educational Research Journal* 33(6), 927–942. DOI: 10.1080/01411920701657033.

Merkies, K., McKechnie, M.J. and Zakrajsek, E. (2018) Behavioural and physiological responses of therapy horses to mentally traumatized humans. *Applied Animal Behaviour Science* 205, 61–67. DOI: 10.1016/j.applanim.2018.05.019.

Schroeder, K., Arant, M., Hekkert, C. and Protopopova, A. (2023) Exploring the social reinforcing value of brushing in equine-assisted services: a comparative study with food reinforcement. *Human-Animal Interactions* 31 March 2023. Available at: https://www.cabidigitallibrary.org/doi/10.1079/hai.2023.0010 (accessed 14 July 2023).

5 Communicating with "Critters"— Incorporating Small Animals into Animal-assisted Interventions

PATTI ANDERSON*

Doggone Good Coaching, LLC, Plymouth, Minnesota, USA

Abstract

When partnering with "pocket pets" or rabbits in animal-assisted intervention (AAI) work, there are various safety aspects one must consider to ensure a positive experience for both the animals and the humans. Selecting an appropriate AAI animal and providing them with a permanent home, coupled with a comprehensive knowledge of the species, including how to recognize and address their stress responses can help mitigate potential welfare issues. This chapter describes some of these important components and best practices of AAI with "pocket pets" or rabbits in AAI work.

"This is the calmest I have felt in months", crooned a teenager with bright purple hair. They sat cross legged on the carpeted floor in a classroom at an alternative high school, stroking "Glinda", a long-haired Peruvian guinea pig. Glinda was making soft purring noises, a sign that she was very content. There were several other teens sprawled out in various positions on the floor, observing the connection made between their classmate and Glinda, experiencing animal-assisted intervention (AAI) in action! The smallest of animals, such as "pocket pets" or rabbits, can often make a big difference in someone's life. These particular teens were working with the school's social worker who was also an AAI practitioner.

Pocket pets and rabbits are prey animals (as opposed to predators). Since these types of small animals are low on the food chain, they are hard wired to be on high alert at all times. Their main defense is to flee the scene and hide. If that fails, they may feel trapped and go into panic mode: biting, scratching and struggling to escape. Some small animals are so terrified when they feel threatened, they might injure themselves trying to escape, go into shock, or worse.

"Pocket pets" is a general term used to describe small mammals kept as pets. Some of the more common species include gerbils, hamsters, guinea pigs, ferrets, chinchillas, mice, rats, and hedgehogs. Bunnies vary in size from the tiny 2 lb (0.9 kg) dwarf rabbit to the Flemish or continental giants which can weigh up to 25 lb (11.34 kg).

AAI practitioners who wish to partner with these types of smaller prey animals need to embrace these two words as their "mantra": *due diligence*! It is important to have an in-depth knowledge of the smaller species an AAI practitioner might work with, meeting the physical and emotional needs for that individual animal. A trusting relationship needs to be established and maintained through regular positive interactions with the AAI animal, no matter what their size, learning how to communicate effectively with them. This human–animal connection is at the heart of having a safe experience for the animal and humans alike.

Let's take a closer look behind the scenes of this actual AAI session with Glinda and explore what it takes to ensure her physical and emotional well-being, which will extend to also mitigating safety issues for the people she works with.

*Siberpa@aol.com

© CAB International 2024. *Animal-assisted Interventions: Recognizing and Mitigating Potential Welfare Challenges* (ed. L.R. Kogan)
DOI: 10.1079/9781800622616.0005

For comparison's sake, let's imagine someone that has never gone bowling before. It looks fairly easy through a beginner's eyes; just grab a ball, roll it down the lane and knock over some pins. How hard could it be? Beginner bowlers quickly learn that there is a specific hand grip, a certain size and weight of ball to use, timed footwork, in addition to many other factors involved.

First impressions of someone not familiar with what is involved with an AAI session might have observed Glinda in the classroom and assumed that this experience looked fairly easy to create. They might surmise that the practitioner had just grabbed a guinea pig from a pet store, then subsequently brought them to school to create the "warm fuzzy" moment they were observing.

Here is an overview of the general process and due diligence for incorporating a small animal like Glinda into AAI work:

1. Glinda was mindfully selected from a reputable breeder. Glinda was only 6 weeks old, but was already the most outgoing in her litter. Peruvians may purr when they feel safe, another way to assess an interaction.
2. There were other adult female pigs at Glinda's new home, so a larger cage was required to accommodate the herd.
3. An exotic animal veterinarian completed a wellness check on Glinda.
4. Several times a day over many months, Glinda was handled for brief periods of time.
5. She was introduced to a variety of people when visitors stopped by, including children.
6. Glinda was exposed to new sensations and experiences in order to desensitize her. These included: (i) different scents (including fur from other animals); (ii) new sounds; (iii) various types of clothing; (iv) typical and atypical movements people might make; (iv) hand feeding; and (vii) sitting in a soft bed or held against someone's shoulder, just to name a few.
7. The crate, used for when the cage was being cleaned or while she was out travelling in it, was her "happy place", as she received special treats in that space.
8. Grooming sessions were done on a regular basis using positive techniques, including handling of her feet, ears, and mouth area. Cheek rubs are a favorite for guinea pigs and assists in desensitizing them to being touched on the mouth.

9. Glinda practiced traveling in her crate to pet stores to safely view dogs and other pets at a distance while eating treats.
10. Since they are herd animals (not all pocket pets are), Glinda always traveled with a senior guinea pig as her buddy, which had a calming effect on her.
11. Glinda benefited from practicing short visits in a controlled setting by traveling to the homes of friends and family members.
12. After 10 months of training Glinda for AAI work, the practitioner prepared her for the Pet Partners (a national non-profit therapy animal organization) evaluation. They passed (Glinda *and* the AAI practitioner), becoming a registered team.
13. Glinda started visiting! She trusted her AAI partner to know her threshold for doing AAI work and keeping her safe by engaging in proactive handling skills.

There was a lot involved with Glinda's therapy journey, but paramount was keeping her best interests in mind.

Well-intended people acquire pocket pets or rabbits for their home every day without researching their basic needs. Their lack of knowledge usually results in the animal having behavior problems, health issues, or both. Some of the common mistakes people make with pocket pets or rabbits are: (i) having inadequate housing; (ii) irregular cleaning of the environment; (iii) improper handling (or the animal not being handled at all); (iv) a resident pet stalking the animal; (v) a poor diet; (vi) lack of enrichment opportunities; (vii) lack of veterinarian involvement; (viii) living without other animals of the same species (again, many are herd animals); or (ix) inadequate grooming.

To get a sense of how many pocket pets and rabbits are typically advertised as needing a new home, a quick peek at the Internet revealed listings within 10 miles of my home for: 17 guinea pigs, three mice, 16 rats, 12 hamsters, eight rabbits, two ferrets and one hedgehog. By the next week, those animals would likely all be gone and more would take their place. The reasons listed for re-homing these animals included "can't afford", and "no time for this pet", at the top of the list, in addition to a long litany of other reasons.

"Tanzy", a tawny-colored lion head rabbit, ended up in an animal shelter after she was abandoned in the snow and rescued by one of the neighbors.

Tanzy was ultimately adopted by an occupational therapist at a long-term care facility who wanted to incorporate an AAI program. It was soon obvious that Tanzy not only liked people, she loved them! Later that year, after the occupational therapist established a trusting relationship with her rabbit, Tanzy (visited only on certain days) became an integral part of the activities program at that facility.

The occupational therapist knew Tanzy's stress signs, which included measuring her respiration rate by counting the number of nose twitches in a set amount of time during a visit and comparing that number to the rate her nose twitched when relaxing at home. She was a proactive handler who made sure Tanzy enjoyed the work that they did together.

Tanzy's story had a positive ending; yet many pocket pets and rabbits have a different ending. Assess your own situation before unintentionally becoming a part of the perpetual "revolving door" for pocket pets or rabbits being re-homed. Do your homework and research the pros and cons of inviting whichever smaller species interests you into your life and AAI work.

If you feel ready to implement an AAI program that partners with either a pocket pet or rabbit, I have listed some best practices below.

Safeguarding the Environment

- Arrange the AAI session to take place indoors. Birds of prey or loose pets may put the animal at risk. If the animal gets loose, it will be difficult to recover them if outside.
- Post a "Do Not Enter" sign on the door during the AAI session.
- Insist that dogs or cats should not be at the facility that day, or at a minimum are secured in a crate behind a locked door during the AAI session.
- Connect with the designated staff person, scope out the physical layout, and ascertain who is in charge of the participants.
- Assess the temperature of the room that will be utilized, as pocket pets and rabbits are very susceptible to overheating or cold drafts.
- Staff should be present during the AAI session. If there is an emergency, practitioners need to be responsible for their animal and not for the participants.

- Small prey animals are alert to bright lights, loud noises, or sudden movements. Lower the lights if possible and limit any noise from an open window, music soundtrack, etc.

Handler Responsibilities

- Transport the AAI animal in a hard-shell crate, such as a top-loading cat crate, rather than pulling them out of a "tunnel"-type carrier. The animal needs to have adequate room to move around in it, places to hide, and an attached water bottle.
- Utilize a well-fitting harness and leash that the animal is accustomed to in order to help prevent them from getting loose in the room and hurting themselves.
- The animal should always have access to a "hidey hole" where they can choose to go if they are feeling stressed or threatened.
- Instruct the participants, before introducing the animal, on how to interact with them. "Show and tell" them how to pet the animal. Ahead of time, practitioners may use a stuffed animal representing that species for participants to practice petting.
- Depending on the nature of the participants, utilize a screening tool for anyone who might have a history of animal abuse, impulse-control issues or have difficulty following instructions. Discuss these participants with the staff for options that prioritize the AAI animal's safety and well-being.
- The staff should screen the participants for allergies, either to the species or their food (such as Timothy hay, a staple for guinea pigs and rabbits). If the animal is on the floor or on furniture, a barrier such as a fleece blanket is used to protect an unsuspecting person entering the room later from having an allergic reaction to any fur strands that may remain.
- In a medical setting, a staff person should be present in order to assist with a barrier for the bed or chair in each room. They will know the standard precautions for each patient, and assist with managing any medical equipment.
- Protect the animal and humans involved from any zoonotic transmissions (diseases spread between animals and humans) by grooming the animal before an AAI session, checking for mites, skin issues, etc. Regular

veterinarian checks, including fecal samples, are recommended.

- Follow the guidelines for appropriate hand hygiene. Everyone involved with the AAI session should either wash their hands with soap and water, or apply hand sanitizer before and after they touch the animal.

The key to recognizing and mitigating potential welfare issues with pocket pets or rabbits is to have extensive knowledge of the species and their stress responses. It is also imperative to develop a trusting relationship with each individual animal, applying best practices to every AAI session. Lastly, and perhaps most important, remember that we have much to learn from animals; be open to hearing what they can teach us.

Keep in mind that "We have more to learn from animals, than animals have to learn from us". (Anthony Douglas Williams; Williams, n.d.).

Reference

Williams, A.D. (n.d.) Anthony D. Williams. AZ Quotes. Available at: https://www.azquotes.com/quote/832706 (accessed 14 March 2023).

6 The Therapy Animal's Bill of Rights

ANN R. HOWIE*

Human-Animal Solutions, PLLC, Olympia, Washington, USA

Abstract

This chapter examines each point of The Therapy Animal's Bill of Rights. It encourages readers to explore ways to incorporate the points into their relationship and interactions with their animals—not just during work time, but also during play and everyday-life activities.

The Therapy Animal's Bill of Rights© (Howie, 2015)

As a therapy animal, I have the right to a handler who:

- obtains my consent to participate in the work;
- provides gentle training to help me understand what I'm supposed to do;
- is considerate of my perception of the world;
- helps me adapt to the work environment;
- guides the client, staff, and visitors to interact with me appropriately;
- focuses on me as much as the client, staff, and visitors;
- pays attention to my non-verbal cues;
- takes action to reduce my stress;
- supports me during interactions with the client;
- protects me from overwork by limiting the length of sessions;
- gives me ways to relax after sessions;
- provides a well-rounded life with nutritious food, physical and mental exercise, social time, and activities beyond work; and
- respects my desire to retire from work when I think it is time.

The Therapy Animal's Bill of Rights (Howie, 2015) has been so well received that it is being used internationally as a guide and pledge for therapy animal handlers. It grew from my personal experience spanning nearly 30 years' training dogs and working with therapy animals in human healthcare and mental health settings. The brief point-by-point explanations here reflect my experiences; I encourage you to find and practice your own embodiment of each point.

Unfortunately, it took me a few years to recognize that therapy animal welfare is an issue. This happened when my second therapy dog became severely ill. After I stopped her work, she recovered and happily lived *years* instead of the few months that our compassionate and knowledgeable veterinarian predicted. That experience weighs heavily on me still. It brought me face to face with the fact that therapy animal welfare starts, proceeds, and ends with the handler (i.e. me). I now remind myself frequently of my responsibility to be alert and responsive to my animal's communication—at home, at work, at the veterinarian, at play—always. Animals communicate constantly. It is up to us to listen (Fig. 6.1).

To emphasize the critical role of the handler, each point of The Therapy Animal's Bill of Rights starts with this phrase, "As a therapy animal, I have the right to a handler who . . . ." To improve the reader's flow, this phrase is not repeated with each point that follows.

As a Therapy Animal, I Have the Right to a Handler Who:

Obtains my consent to participate in the work

I ask for my therapy animal's consent not just once every 2 years during recredentialing, not

*Humananimalsolutions@comcast.net

DOI: 10.1079/9781800622616.0006

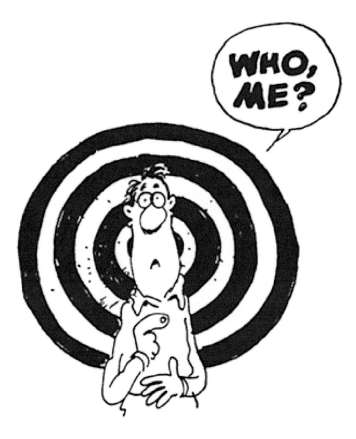

Fig. 6.1. It is up to us to listen to animals.

just at the beginning of a session, but constantly throughout each session. I get his consent or denial by watching his expressive behavior (Figs 6.2 and 6.3).

I have found Suzanne Clothier's Elemental Questions (Clothier, 2014) provide an excellent framework for questions to ask and ways to listen for my animal's answers.

Provides gentle training to help me understand what I'm supposed to do

It is important to me to be respectful of my animal companions, while working, playing, or resting. Maintaining an attitude of respect for my animals includes using training methods that avoid coercion. In my interactions with my animals, including training, I want to help them feel safe and competent, feelings which grow from knowing what to do. To this end, I identify my expectations of their behavior (in sessions and at home) and gently/respectfully train toward those expectations, thus helping them gain competence (Fig. 6.4).

Is considerate of my perception of the world

Animals *hear* different frequencies from those humans hear (Fig. 6.5a), so I avoid the assumption that just because I don't hear something there is nothing to be heard.

Animals *see* different colors from those humans see (Fig. 6.5b), so I intentionally choose colors in my work environment that my animals can see.

Animals are a different height from humans, so their literal line of sight differs from what we see. Further, depending on where their eyes are placed on their heads, their field of vision may

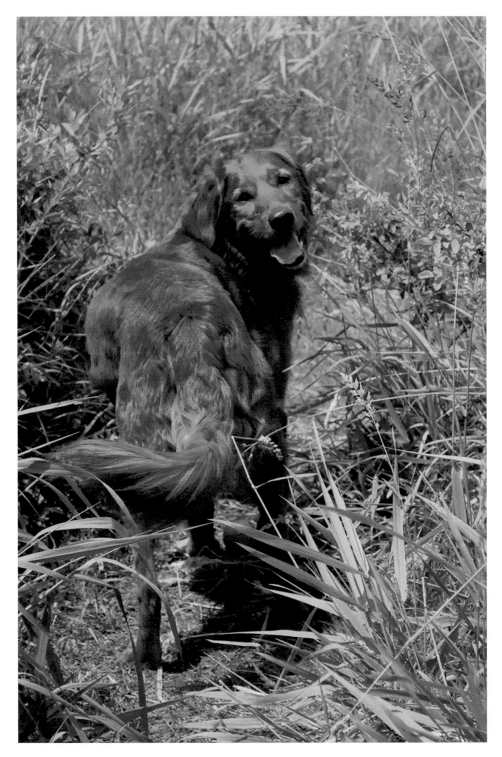

Fig. 6.2. This dog happily consents.

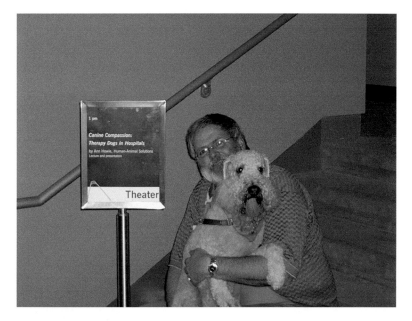

Fig. 6.3. This dog is hot, tired, and about to be cranky. He has withdrawn consent.

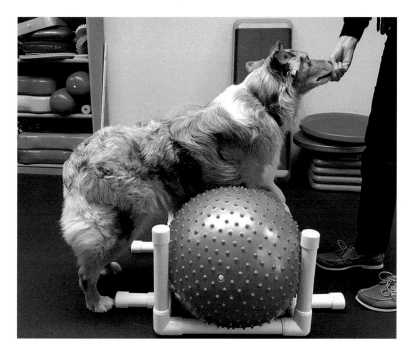

Fig. 6.4. This dog is learning how to appropriately get closer to clients.

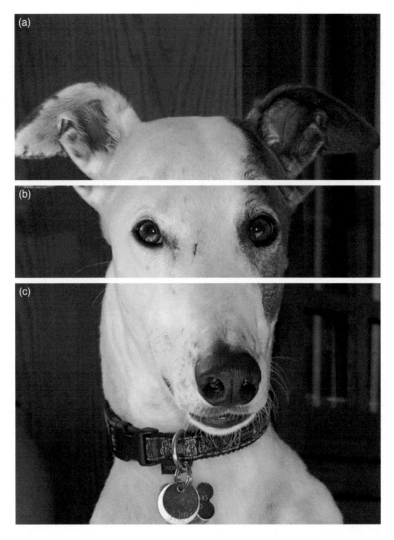

Fig. 6.5. Animals hear (a), see (b), and perceive scent (c) differently from humans.

include far more of the periphery than does mine. I frequently kneel to look at things from my dog's perspective.

Animals perceive *scent* differently from humans (Fig. 6.5c). I remind myself that if *I* can smell a strong scent, it may be overpowering to my animal. (And I think I am rather glad that I can't identify all the odors that are accessible to them.)

In combination with attentiveness to my animal's perceptions and senses, I watch his behavior during time with and between clients, and I adjust my sessions accordingly to protect him.

Helps me adapt to the work environment

Because my human lifestyle takes me to a variety of locations, and because my animal does not have the same access or frequency of exposure, things which are commonplace to me may be disturbing to my animal. I again remain watchful of my animal's behavior. If I notice an unusual response (approach, avoidance, or hesitation) to something in the work environment (Fig. 6.6), I make note, change what's going on in the moment to reduce the effect on my animal, and continue to assess my

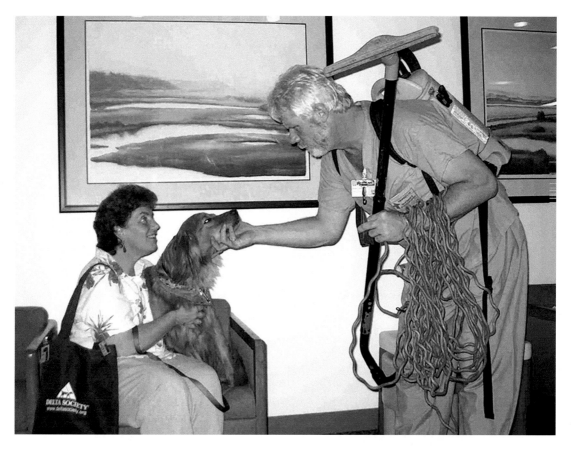

Fig. 6.6. Common work environments can present challenges to animals.

animal's response. If my animal finds something aversive, I choose not to train for desensitization. Instead, I do not place my animal into that situation. This means that my *animal* (not me) gets to choose what is pleasant and unpleasant, and I get to adjust accordingly.

Guides the client, staff, and visitors to interact with me appropriately

As Pet Partners says so eloquently, "You are your animal's best advocate" (YAYABA). My animal depends on me to create a session that is respectful of him (Fig. 6.7). I use therapeutic interventions to help clients adjust the way they interact with my animal, based on my observation of his response. Without continuous observation and responding in

the moment, I will fail in advocating for my animal. It is not good enough to make assumptions based on his past responses; I must remain in the present.

Focuses on me as much as the client, staff, and visitors

Even while the client is the focus of a session, my focus is on my animal just as much as or more than the client. This means that I practice at splitting my attention between the client and my animal. And for animal welfare, my animal comes first (Fig. 6.8). By putting my animal's safety first, the people around us will also be safe because I have not pushed him into a situation where he needs to strongly express his opinion (either negative or overly positive) or retaliate.

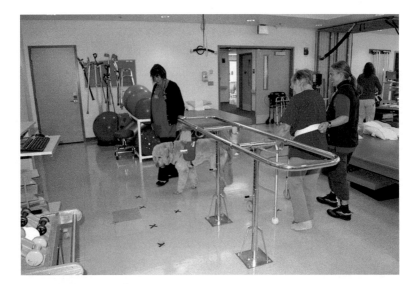

Fig. 6.7. This handler chooses a follow-the-leader interaction in this situation.

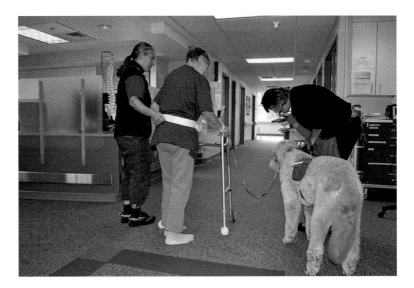

Fig. 6.8. This handler takes time to assure her dog's readiness.

Pays attention to my non-verbal cues

Here's the central importance of observation: if I don't see something, I can't take action. Part of my centering process before a client session begins includes tuning into my animal. This helps me avoid paying so much attention to the client that I miss what my animal is saying (Fig. 6.9).

Takes action to reduce my stress

Noticing is only part of what's needed. Not only must I observe, but I must also act in support of what I observe (Fig. 6.10). This sometimes means shortening a session or adjusting the session for my animal's welfare. I keep a client-free zone in my office: a comfy dog bed in a familiar and

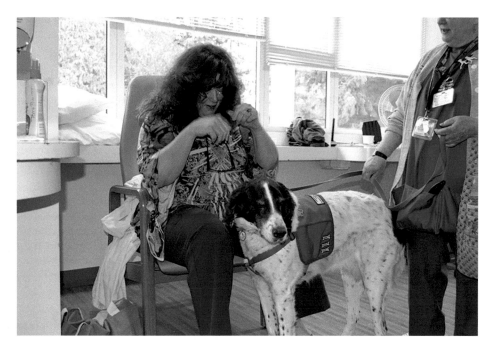

Fig. 6.9. This dog is starting to show stress by turning away.

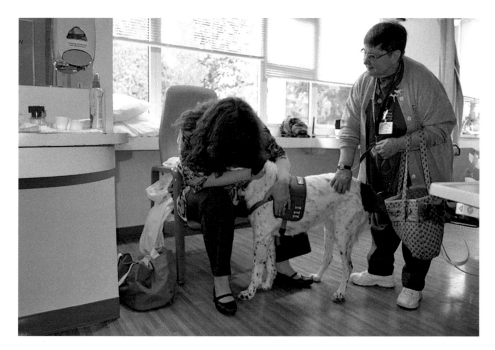

Fig. 6.10. This handler touched her dog in support, then gently withdrew her dog from the interaction.

---

restful crate located around a wall from the treatment area. I allow my dog to be off leash during sessions so that he can leave the client and go into that area of his own volition. I discuss this possibility with clients initially so that I have something to refer to if/when my dog chooses self-care over client care.

Supports me during interactions with the client

Part of my initial client assessment and education about animal-assisted therapy includes a discussion of what might happen during sessions. "What might happen" includes my dog's behavior as well as my behavior, toward both my dog and the client. If it is therapeutically indicated, I might ask if the client notices my dog panting (for example). Together we might identify various courses of action to take care of my dog's needs (like refreshing the water bowl or opening a window for some fresh air). We might wonder why my dog is panting and explore whether the client has had similar experiences, relating the dog's experience to the client's and making parallels regarding self-care. Within the session, I speak conversationally, touch, watch, and/or move close to him to offer additional support (Fig. 6.11).

Protects me from overwork by limiting the length of sessions

My animals don't work every day, nor do they work 8 hours a day. When I'm working with my animal, I also make sure to insert breaks into the day (that I might not do just for myself) (Fig. 6.12).

Gives me ways to relax after sessions

A friend of mine in Japan calls this "recovery" time. Recovery time is made up of what my animal thinks is relaxing (not what is relaxing for me) (Fig. 6.13). To one of my dogs, a special food snack was essential. Another dog preferred a quiet walk in the woods. A horse loved to gallop. A cat insisted on unbothered nap time at home. Whatever it is, I incorporate that time into my animal's workday to assure my animal's welfare.

Provides a well-rounded life with nutritious food, physical and mental exercise, social time, and activities beyond work

A well-rounded life can be closely related to the prior point, yet it is also separate. The sport of canine nosework is something my dogs relish (Fig. 6.14). Using their brains (along with their noses) helps

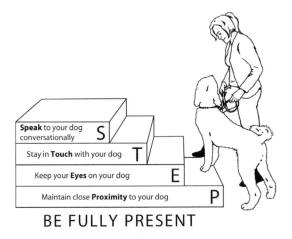

Fig. 6.11. The STEPs of teamwork (Howie, 2015).

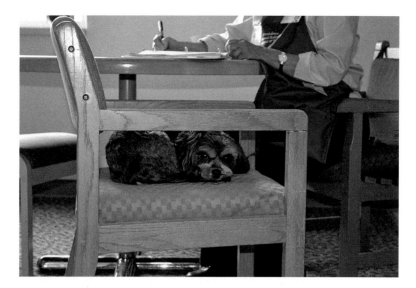

Fig. 6.12. This dog gets a break while her handler completes documentation.

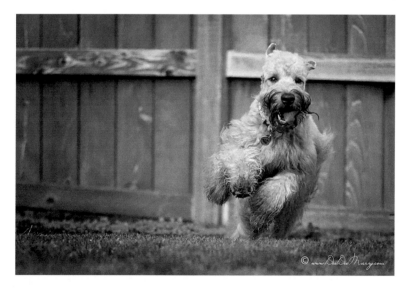

Fig. 6.13. This dog enjoys a romp in wet grass after work.

provide balance to the pressures they experience from working. There are numerous dog sport options for non-work time, and other fun options for other species. Further, physical conditioning is a key component of good health, and my dogs and I delight in sharing physical fitness training. Some of my dogs have craved to play with dog friends and others have not. Whatever it is my animals relish, I prioritize engaging in these activities to assure that they have a well-rounded lifestyle.

Respects my desire to retire from work when I think it is time

I remember returning to my car after a session with one of my dogs and crying into the steering wheel

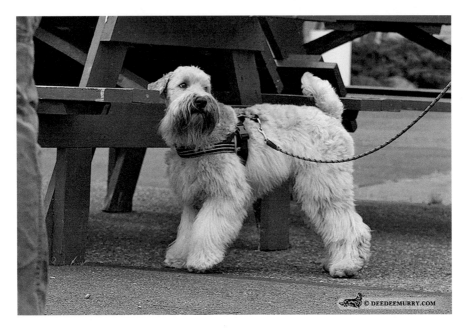

Fig. 6.14. This dog gives an alert after finding the target scent in nosework.

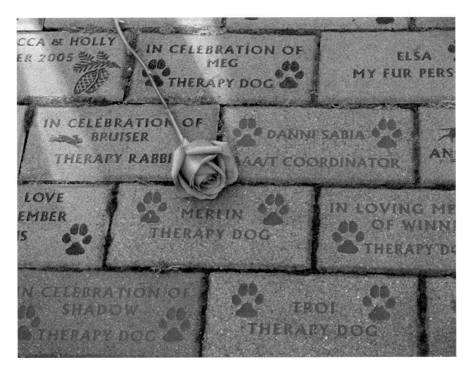

Fig. 6.15. Pavers honoring the work of therapy dogs.

A.R. Howie

because I realized that it had been my dog's last working day. I loved the work, and so did that dog, but his body wasn't able to maintain the rigors of the work. So he was retired on that day. As hard as that was for me, he came first. He, like other retired therapy animals, went on to enjoy a retirement but their contribution to the lives of others is not forgotten (Fig. 6.15).

I hope these personal examples have given you some ideas about how The Therapy Animal's Bill of Rights might apply to you and your animal. It is my hope that we all incorporate these aspects into our work with our therapy animals, as well as our everyday life with our companion animals. They will thank us for it.

Discussion questions

1. Which of the points in The Therapy Animal's Bill of Rights is the most challenging for you? Why?
2. How do you think The Therapy Animal's Bill of Rights applies to non-working companion animals in your household?

References

Clothier, S. (2014) Presentation for the reflected relationship seminar. August 2014. St. Johnsville, New York.

Howie, A.R. (2015) *Teaming With Your Therapy Dog*. Purdue University Press, West Lafayette, Indiana. DOI: 10.2307/j.ctv15wxpvx.

7 Trauma-informed Interspecies Social Justice in AAI

Sᴀʀᴀʜ Sᴄʜʟᴏᴛᴇ*

EQUUSOMA® Horse–Human Trauma Recovery, Guelph, Ontario, Canada

Abstract

Animal-assisted interventions (AAIs) often provide meaningful psychosocial opportunities for people facing trauma and marginalization. Without applying a trauma and social justice lens to the animals involved, AAIs risk repeating harmful dynamics that undermine the experience for all involved. This chapter outlines some examples of re-enactments that can unfold as a result of anthropocentrism and speciesism to reinforce the importance of prioritizing the welfare of both human and animal participants.

Social justice refers to the process of identifying and dismantling barriers that disproportionately impact certain groups, resulting in systemic experiences of oppression, unmet needs, adversity, and disparities in terms of health, welfare, and well-being. These disparities usually reflect power and control dynamics that are rooted in layers of privilege, discrimination, or implicit bias that benefit members of certain groups at the expense of members of other groups. A common example is where buildings, public spaces, facilities, and equipment are designed with able-bodied individuals in mind, which makes it difficult for people with various medical, physical, or mental health needs to participate in society in an equal way. From this standpoint, what is disabling is not their condition but the lack of universal design, accommodations, and non-judgmental acceptance that would facilitate their inclusion.

A related phenomenon is that of inspiration porn (Young, 2012), referring to the portrayal of individuals who are facing various adversities or barriers as inspirational to those who are not facing those particular challenges. The insidious message of inspiration porn is that success is ultimately a matter of having the right attitude, regardless of the number of systemic barriers that may legitimately be exacerbating their difficulties or may even be (re)traumatizing. This simultaneously objectifies the oppressed individual for the more privileged viewer's gratification while absolving the latter from any responsibility related to their participation in a system that supports their comfort at the expense of others.

Anthropocentrism in AAI

The field of animal-assisted interventions (AAIs) is not immune to issues of social injustice and inspiration porn. Many AAIs provide much-needed support to underserved and/or marginalized populations in an effort to reduce disparities and facilitate a sense of inclusion. Such programs often receive media exposure and widespread acclaim for how inspiring they are. However, these same programs may occur at the expense of the animals involved. For instance, many AAI programs are designed for people facing trauma, stress, tragedy, discrimination, exploitation, barriers, or a lack of resources related to early adversity, health, racism, ableism, ageism, sexism, colonialism, capitalism, cis-heteronormativity, education, socio-economic status, and other risk factors. However, in spite of being trauma informed and/or social justice focused for the human client, some such programs may nonetheless be founded in anthropocentrism and speciesism, where animals are objectified,

*info@equusoma.com

DOI: 10.1079/9781800622616.0007

commodified, and serve as gratification of human needs, sometimes at the animal's expense.

Social and mainstream media are replete with examples of animals involved in programs that are intended for human benefit. Sometimes there is a discrepancy between the glowing narrative and comments that extol the virtues of the human–animal bond, and the accompanying images or videos that depict animals showing signs of annoyance, appeasement, aversion, pain, or discomfort, which are either overtly disregarded or simply not recognized by those offering and receiving the interventions and by those voicing their endorsement. In these cases, AAIs offer a different kind of inspiration porn, where animals are glorified as cure-alls for those who struggle, which provides a feel-good justification for AAIs that celebrates human benevolence and good intentions towards the less fortunate, while simultaneously distancing the viewers, those offering, and those benefiting from AAIs from any responsibility in their participation in a system that exists at the potential cost of the animals.

Role Reversals

Of course, many AAI programs follow protocols and principles that aim to ensure the welfare of both the humans and the animals involved, as evidenced in this book. However, when these protocols are not followed, the result can be an unfortunate re-enactment in terms of who is committing harm ("perpetrator"), who is helping ("rescuer"), and who is needing help ("victim"), in accordance with the drama triangle (Karpman, 1968), repeating similar power dynamics to those experienced by the human clients in the first place. For instance, consider a situation where a person leading an AAI has unresolved trauma that results in a pattern of codependence where they help others at their own expense ("rescuer"), so as to make up for the actions or inactions of the people and systems that have caused harm ("perpetrator"), which may inadvertently remove agency and self-determination from the client who is seen as suffering and in need of help ("victim"). The "rescuer" feels empowered for contributing to society, in part because helping was a way to prevent harm and avoid feeling powerless as a child, and being seen as altruistic and kind may also assuage underlying shame related to a core message that they had to earn love by being good and useful to others. This underlying pattern of appeasement may

make the person leading AAIs less likely to recognize how the animal may be appeasing and/or overriding as well. In that case, the roles in the triangle shift, where the "rescuer" and the "victim" (however unintentionally) adopt the role of "perpetrator" of harm towards the new "victim", the animal.

Having a human client engage in an activity that benefits them over the needs of the animal places both in an untenable position. If the client does not recognize the re-enactment right away and later realizes that the animal is facing something similar to what they themselves experienced, they may: (i) either feel appalled or guilty for being complicit in that dynamic; (ii) be ashamed for now being in a similar position of "power over" as their abuser, even if involuntarily; (iii) resume suppressing their own needs after taking the risk to express them (especially if they had codependent patterns to start with); and (iv) face a double bind about whether or not to express these feelings, as well as any anger and distrust they might now have, towards the person leading the AAI for setting up the situation. The outcome reinforces a felt sense of unsafety in relationship for both the human client and the animal, which undermines the goals and intentions of the AAI.

Magic Unicorn Syndrome

A related phenomenon is what I call "magic unicorn syndrome" (Schlote, 2019a, Schlote, 2019b), also known as "unicorn-assisted therapy" (Lundgren, 2019). This refers to the objectification, commodification, and/or anthropomorphizing of equines as magical beings or co-therapists, and the implicit or unconscious expectations that may result. Historically, the idea of equines as co-therapists evolved as a counter-response to approaches and programs that used animals as tools without much regard for their own trauma histories, patterns, temperaments, and needs. Referring to equines as co-therapists or co-facilitators usually reflects an intention to acknowledge their sentience, individuality, and agency. However, referring to both the clients and the animals in AAI as participants avoids the pitfalls of anthropomorphizing and objectification that can occur when applying a human-based career label to another species. Additional reasons for not referring to animals as co-therapists or co-facilitators include:

- human professionals generally perform their role with an awareness of many layers of information and expectations related to scope of practice, legislation, ethics, and/or standards, which animals are incapable of understanding and are not held to in the same way;

- human professionals have a duty of care to attend to the animals' needs in the experience, to ensure that their involvement does not negatively impact them (do no harm) and at best is beneficial to them (do good), just as they do the human client, whereas animals do not have this same duty of care;
- human professionals cannot simply walk away from a client mid-intervention, whereas an animal—if its sentience and agency are supported—could; and
- an animal cannot act as a therapist or facilitator independently without a human professional present (what makes the intervention "therapy" or "experiential learning" is the presence of a human professional operating within a specific scope), no matter how therapeutic or instructive unstructured time spent with animals may be.

The rationale for avoiding referring to horses as "healers" is similar. Some humans who call themselves healers may be engaging in a form of spiritual or communal narcissism, where they derive a sense of grandiosity at having special powers that are unique and needed by others, and reinforce the idea that they are more helpful, wise, evolved, and therefore better positioned to save or rescue others or the world (Ferrer and Vickery, 2018; Ingraham, 2019; Vonk and Visser, 2020; Beeden, 2021). This underlying belief system may be concealed under a veil of benevolence. These patterns risk fostering a sense of dependence on the healer and undermine the client's agency, inner locus of control, and self-determination in terms of their own healing. In addition, the concept of healer in Western society may at times reflect cultural appropriation by White people of methods that belong to various Indigenous groups or other cultural or spiritual communities, sometimes known as "plastic shamanism" (Mayo, 1991; Aldred, 2000). The Western phenomenon of spiritual narcissism also provides a foundation upon which egoic "guru culture" perpetuates harm through the distorted misuse of healing or shamanic practices (Kaufman, 2021).

When horses are painted in a similar brushstroke, there can be a similar risk of expectation by the professional and/or the client that the horse has magical powers that will heal the client. This can result in its behaviour (even its stress responses) being misinterpreted as having healing intentions or messages for the human client, while simultaneously not addressing what may be generating said stress responses. There may also be secondary gains in calling a horse a healer: doing so may generate revenue by appealing to those for whom the idea of being healed or rescued by another being fills a need that went unmet by unresponsive, unreliable, or unsafe adults when they were little. This runs the risk of a re-enactment where the equine is pressured or coerced into providing a healing experience (to ensure that the client is satisfied, pays, and returns), and where the human client is set up for potential disappointment or harm if the animal does not offer such an experience. If the professional is also driven by a need to be liked or by a need to rescue so that the human client leaves feeling good, this can further contribute to these unconscious dynamics.

Certainly, many programs that refer to equines as co-therapists, co-facilitators, or healers are operating in ways that are ethical and show integrity and awareness related to these factors. That said, referring to animals as participants in AAIs does not diminish their significant contributions, many of which may defy explanation in terms of how astute, attuned, profound, beneficial, and therapeutic their involvement may be. It merely acknowledges that they are individuals first and foremost, which affords them more freedom to show up in whatever way is authentic to them in any given moment without the confines of particular expectations or obligations associated with human role labels.

Incongruent Congruence

Animals can provide opportunities for humans to experience safe touch, co-regulation, explore boundaries, and experience a sense of inner congruence, where their thoughts, feelings, bodily sensations, and actions align. However, an incongruent double standard exists when the same is not afforded to the animals involved. For instance, an AAI facilitator may be well intentioned in inviting a client to reach out and touch or pet an animal to explore sensory grounding, and may then describe the subsequent sense of calm in the client as evidence of co-regulation, further legitimizing the experience. However, if said facilitator also subtly blocks the animal from moving away from the client's touch, and the animal simply tolerates the experience from a place of appeasement or shutdown, co-regulation would not be a congruent explanation for why the client feels calmer or a sense of enjoyment in that moment. This can also be the case if an animal is off-leash or "at liberty": depending on its training or past experiences, an animal might not move away if it feels uncomfortable, and may simply check out mentally, freeze, or appease in place, giving the illusion of consent or willingness. Some facilitators may even explain that the animal has the ability to move away if it chooses, implying that the animal staying is always by choice, when this may not be the case. People who also responded similarly when uncomfortable or unsafe may feel shame or subtly blamed for what happened to them because they, too, did not choose to leave. Alternatively, a horse approaching or 'joining up' with a client in a round pen may be a sign of social engagement and connection, but it may also be an artifact of being isolated away from its herd, opting to engage because it would rather do so than be alone, something that the client may have had to resort to themselves at times. A client who also engages in these survival responses might not feel truly seen or heard if the person leading the AAI does not recognize these similar responses playing out in the animal. Finally, co-regulation requires that one nervous system is in a state that is conducive to inducing calm and connection in the other nervous system (Kain and Terrell, 2018). If a human client experiences calm, joy, or exuberance while engaging with or touching a shutdown or appeasing animal, this may be due to being away from their problematic circumstances, out in nature, experiencing novelty, the presence of the person leading the AAI, or other variables—as opposed to co-regulation.

AAIs have great potential in supporting trauma and social injustice-affected populations. Given that domesticated animals exist in human-controlled environments, it is essential that those offering AAIs dismantle systemic structures and beliefs while also addressing their own implicit biases and trauma patterns with compassion. Both human and animal bodies can have a history of experiencing harm in relationships, and their healing and liberation can be mutually experienced in relationship as well, provided that such a framework guides the process, even if the human is the identified client.

Bibliography

Aldred, L. (2000) Plastic shamans and astroturf sundances: new age commercialization of Native American spirituality. *American Indian Quarterly* 24(3), 329–352. DOI: 10.1353/aiq.2000.0001.

Beeden, K. (2021) How to spot spiritual narcissists. *Medium,* September 29. Available at: https://medium.com/@katiabeeden/fake-healers-are-real-b272ac3877c (accessed 20 January 2023).

Ferrer, J.N. and Vickery, W.Z. (2018) Transpersonal psychology and the spiritual but not religious movement: beyond spiritual narcissism in a postsecular age. In: Parsons, W.B. (ed.) *Being Spiritual but Not Religious: Past, Present, Future(s)*. Routledge, London, pp. 219–235. DOI: 10.4324/9781315107431.

Ingraham, P. (2019) *Healer Syndrome*, November 16. Available at: https://www.painscience.com/articles/healer-syndrome.php (accessed 22 January 2023).

Kain, K.L. and Terrell, S.J. (2018) *Nurturing Resilience: Helping Clients Move Forward from Developmental Trauma*. North Atlantic Books, Berkeley, California.

Karpman, S. (1968) Fairy tales and script drama analysis. *Transactional Analysis Bulletin* 7(26), 39–43.

Kaufman, S.B. (2021) The science of spiritual narcissism. *Scientific American,* January 11. Available at: https://www.scientificamerican.com/article/the-science-of-spiritual-narcissism/ (accessed 30 January 2023).

Levine, P.A. (1997) *Waking the Tiger: Healing Trauma*. North Atlantic Books, Berkeley, California.

Levine, P.A. (2010) *In an Unspoken Voice: How the Body Releases Trauma and Restores Goodness*. North Atlantic Books, Berkeley, California.

Lundgren, K. (2019) Unicorn assisted therapy. *MiMer Centre Blog,* July 19. Available at: https://www.mimercentre.org/index.php/blog/unicorn-assisted-therapy (accessed 20 January 2023).

Mayo, L. (1991) Appropriation and the plastic shaman: Winnetou's snake oil show from Wigwam City. *Canadian Theatre Review* 68, 54–55. DOI: 10.3138/ctr.68.017.

Schlote, S.M. (2019a) Pseudoscience: a brief rant. *EQUUSOMA® Tiger Talk,* June 28. Available at: https://equusoma.com/pseudoscience-a-brief-rant/ (accessed 8 January 2023).

Schlote, S.M. (2019b) Security in connection and co-regulation: safeguarding the horse from traumatic re-enactments in EQUUSOMA. In: Parent, I. (ed.) *A Horse is a Horse, of Course: Compendium from the Third International Symposium for Equine Welfare and Wellness*. Createspace Independent Publishing Platform, Scotts Valley, California, pp. 215–238.

Vonk, R. and Visser, A. (2020) An exploration of spiritual superiority: the paradox of self-enhancement. *European Journal of Social Psychology* 51(1), 152–165. DOI: 10.1002/ejsp.2721.

Young, S. (2012) We're not here for your inspiration. *The Drum,* July 2. Available at: https://www.abc.net.au/news/2012-07-03/young-inspiration-porn/4107006 (accessed 20 January 2023).

8 Recognizing and Mitigating Potential Welfare Challenges During Equine-assisted Services for Autistic Youth

B. Caitlin Peters[1]* and Temple Grandin[2]

[1]Temple Grandin Equine Center, Colorado State University, Fort Collins, Colorado, USA; [2]Colorado State University, Fort Collins, Colorado, USA

Abstract

While equine-assisted services can often be mutually beneficial for both horses and humans, there are several welfare considerations unique to this population. This chapter outlines seven intervention strategies to mitigate potential welfare challenges: (i) get to know the youth's communication styles; (ii) equine selection and training; (iii) practice equine safety before introducing the horse; (iv) use a gait belt and contact-guard assist (an assisting person who has one or two hands on the participant's body but provides no other assistance); (v) introduce appropriate replacement behaviors; (vi) introduce consequences for safe and unsafe behaviors; and (vii) ensure no-horse alternatives are available. The chapter concludes with a case scenario and discussion questions.

Equine-Assisted Services for Autistic Youth

Autism is defined by: (i) impairments in social communication and social interaction; and (ii) restricted or repetitive behaviors, interests, or activities (American Psychiatric Association, 2013). There is wide diversity in how autism manifests differently in each individual, and also among different autistic individuals. Therefore, potential welfare challenges during equine-assisted services (EASs) for autistic youth will vary widely from person to person.

EASs is an umbrella term that is used to describe the many different services that incorporate horses in order to benefit people (Wood *et al.*, 2021). There are over a dozen different EASs that fall into three broad categories: (i) therapy services (occupational therapy, physical therapy, speech-language therapy, psychotherapy, etc.); (ii) horsemanship services (adaptive equestrian sports, adaptive/therapeutic riding, adaptive driving, etc.); and (iii) equine-assisted learning services. Autistic youth may participate in any of these services, but most commonly participate in adaptive riding or therapy services. Autistic individuals are one of the most served populations at facilities that provide EASs (Professional Association of Therapeutic Horsemanship, International, 2020). Research demonstrates EASs can improve a variety of outcomes in autistic youth, including social skills, communication, emotional regulation, and motor skills (McDaniel Peters and Wood, 2017). As an autistic woman (Grandin), I can personally attest to the powerful effect horses had in my life as I was growing up; the barn was a refuge for me away from bullying, I made friends with the other students who went riding, and I learned work skills because I cleaned stalls (Grandin, 2019). While the focus of this book is on potential welfare challenges, it seems important to note that horse–human interactions between autistic youth and horses are often beneficial for both the horses and the humans involved.

*Corresponding author: caiti.peters@colostate.edu

© CAB International 2024. *Animal-assisted Interventions: Recognizing and Mitigating Potential Welfare Challenges* (ed. L.R. Kogan)
DOI: 10.1079/9781800622616.0008

However, this population also presents unique challenges that should be considered in order to ensure the highest welfare for both the horses and the humans involved in the EASs.

Safety Considerations for Autistic Youth Participating in EASs

EASs for any population involve inherent risks. While uncommon, it is possible that participants could be bumped by a horse, stepped on, bitten, or fall off the horse. Furthermore, it is possible that participants could experience fear or nervousness while interacting with such a large animal. Safety concerns specific to autistic youth will vary widely depending on the individual—while some autistic youth may not present any additional safety concerns beyond that of a typical recreational rider, others may. For instance, many autistic youth thrive on routine, and the novelty of interacting with a horse may induce anxiety or fear. Furthermore, the different smells, lighting, dusty air, and textures common in a barn can be difficult for autistic youth who have sensory aversions; I (Peters) once worked with a child who required cotton balls with essential oils in his nose before he could even enter the barn, but once he did, he loved riding his horse. For minimally verbal autistic youth, it may be difficult for the provider to determine if the youth consents to interacting with or riding the horse. Self-regulation difficulties are common in autistic youth (Conner *et al.*, 2021), which can manifest in impulsive behaviors that could present safety challenges, such as running up to the horse, touching the horse's mouth, or dismounting the horse unsafely.

Potential Welfare Concerns for Horses

There are also several potential equine welfare concerns to consider during EASs for autistic youth. Perhaps most commonly, the horse may experience increased stress due to the youth's repetitive behaviors, such as body rocking, hand flapping, or vocalizations that are high-pitched or loud. Furthermore, there is an increased incidence of aggression, irritability, and hyperactivity in autistic youth (Doehring *et al.*, 2014; Kaat *et al.*, 2014), which could present equine welfare challenges if the youth is aggressive toward the horse (i.e. hitting, kicking) or has difficulty staying still while riding. Impaired balance is also common in autistic youth (Stins and Emck, 2018), which

may present welfare challenges in horses due to the increased physical and/or psychological demand of carrying an unbalanced rider.

Intervention Strategies to Mitigate Potential Welfare Challenges

As with EASs for all populations, we highly recommend implementing industry standards for safety and equine welfare put forth by the Professional Association of Therapeutic Horsemanship, International, the American Hippotherapy Association, Inc, the Canadian Therapeutic Riding Association, Riding for the Disabled, or other equivalent body. Above and beyond those recommended standards, we suggest several intervention strategies that can mitigate potential welfare challenges during EASs for autistic youth.

Get to know the youth's communication styles

Prior to introducing a horse, learn how the youth communicates. While many autistic youth communicate verbally, many also communicate via sign language, with a communication device, through their behavior, or through sounds such as whining or squealing. I (Peters) worked with an autistic girl, Carmen, who communicated pleasure through high-pitched squeals and communicated "no" through low grunts or escape behaviors such as running away. Knowing this ahead of time helped me to understand when she did not want to participate in a certain task or when she was enjoying herself.

Equine selection and training

We recommend selecting a horse that is well suited to the autistic individual, taking into consideration the youth's size, motor abilities, and behaviors. Horses in EASs programs are often trained to become desensitized to unbalanced riders, repetitive behaviors (hand flapping, loud vocalizations, etc.), and mounted activities (i.e. mounted basketball, ring toss, etc.). Individual horses vary in their response to these different conditions. In the herd of horses I (Peters) work with, one horse demonstrates behavior indicative of stress in response to an unbalanced rider but not to hand flapping, while another horse with the same training has an opposite reaction (increased stress to hand flapping but not an unbalanced rider). The provider should consider the specific behaviors of each autistic client that could cause increased stress in the horse, and select a horse well matched to that participant.

Practice equine safety before introducing the horse

For some autistic youth, we recommend practicing safe ways to interact with horses before introducing a real horse. Given the concrete-thinking style of most autistic youth, practicing with a life-sized pretend horse (i.e. stuffed horse, mechanical horse, barrel, etc.) can be very helpful. I (Peters) often use a mechanical horse to teach youth how to safely walk near a horse, how to pet a horse's neck, where not to touch a horse, and how to safely mount and dismount. Providing autistic youth with clear expectations prior to interacting with a horse can often decrease anxiety and unsafe behaviors, leading to a more positive experience for both the youth and the horse.

Use a gait belt and contact-guard assist

For autistic youth who demonstrate impulsive or unsafe behaviors, we recommend using a gait belt and maintaining close physical proximity, so that you can stop any potentially unsafe behaviors before they happen. For example, I (Peters) often work with autistic children with a history of elopement (running away). To ensure children do not run while in the barn, I ensure children with a history of elopement wear gait belts and I stay very close to prevent any running before it begins. This strategy can also be effective for other unsafe behaviors such as a desire to touch the horse's face or dismount the horse unsafely.

Introduce appropriate replacement behaviors to autistic youth

In some cases, it is possible to select a horse that is desensitized to potentially problematic behaviors of autistic youth (e.g. hand flapping, vocalizations). However, some behaviors pose a safety risk to either the horse or the participant and simply cannot be tolerated (e.g. pulling the horse's mane, bouncing up and down on the saddle). Teaching autistic youth appropriate replacement behaviors can be an effective intervention strategy to stop unsafe behaviors. Determining an effective replacement behavior requires the provider to consider the function of the unsafe behavior and provide a safe alternative that fulfills the same function. For example, Carmen, an autistic youth, attempted to pull the horse's mane while riding. At first, I (Peters) thought she was seeking increased stability, so I introduced a western saddle with stirrups to provide more stability. She continued to pull the horse's mane, so my next guess was that she liked the feeling of the hair. I tied a fidget to the saddle horn and she immediately stopped grabbing the mane, playing with the fidget instead, as it provided an effective replacement for the sensation of pulling the mane.

Introduce consequences for safe and unsafe behaviors

Positive reinforcement is defined as the introduction of a desired stimulus after a behavior that reinforces the behavior and makes it more likely the behavior will occur again. In the context of EASs, we recommend positively reinforcing youth's safe interactions with horses. One method of positive reinforcement is specific praise, where the provider praises the child for a clearly defined behavior (e.g. "well done Johnny, good job petting the horse on the neck with gentle hands"). Continued interaction with the horse may also serve as an effective reinforcement. Reinforcement should be individualized to each child, based on what is most desirable/pleasing, and therefore effective, for each individual. We also recommend providing clear consequences for unsafe behaviors. For example, in the case of a child who liked to bounce up and down while the horse walked, I (Peters) instructed the horse leader to stop the horse if the child bounced; the horse would not continue walking until he kept his body still. He quickly learned that to ride the horse, which he enjoyed, he could not bounce up and down. A more extreme example may be that of hitting the horse. In my (Peters) practice, if a child hits or kicks the horse, or attempts an unplanned dismount, I immediately safely dismount the child and explain that the consequence for that behavior is that they cannot continue riding today. This consequence both prioritizes the horse's welfare, and teaches the youth that unsafe behaviors are not tolerated around the horse.

Ensure no-horse alternatives are available

While uncommon, it is possible that some autistic youth may be unable to control their unsafe behaviors around horses, in which case it would not be safe for them to participate in EASs. Alternatively, many autistic youth may be able to safely participate in EASs most days, but may also have days where they are particularly dysregulated and unable to safely interact with a horse. We recommend having no-horse alternatives available when needed. As a therapist, I (Peters) often provide occupational therapy in the barn or clinic without interacting with the horse if needed. For adaptive riding, the no-horse alternative may involve barn management activities (cleaning stalls, throwing hay), or learning horsemanship skills with a pretend horse (grooming, rein use, etc.).

Case Example

Carmen is a 7-year-old autistic girl who is minimally verbal, repetitively says "da-da-da" in a high-pitched squeal, and has a history of unsafe behaviors such as running away or jumping off playground equipment. At the evaluation appointment, I learned from her mother that high-pitch squeals were an indication that Carmen was enjoying herself, whereas low-pitch grunts or running away were an indication that Carmen did not want to participate in a given activity. Carmen had a dog at home, and Carmen's mother reported she often tried to pull the dog's tail, and she was concerned that Carmen may also demonstrate unsafe behaviors with the horse.

Discussion questions

1. How would you first introduce Carmen to a horse?
2. What qualities would you consider when selecting a horse for Carmen to ride?

Bibliography

American Psychiatric Association (2013) *Diagnostic and Statistical Manual of Mental Disorders*, 5th edn. American Psychiatric Publishing, Washington, DC. DOI: 10.1176/appi.books.9780890425596.

Conner, C.M., Golt, J., Shaffer, R., Righi, G., Siegel, M. et al. (2021) Emotion dysregulation is substantially elevated in autism compared to the general population: impact on psychiatric services. *Autism Research* 14(1), 169–181. DOI: 10.1002/aur.2450.

Doehring, P., Reichow, B., Palka, T., Phillips, C. and Hagopian, L. (2014) Behavioral approaches to managing severe problem behaviors in children with autism spectrum and related developmental disorders: a descriptive analysis. *Child and Adolescent Psychiatric Clinics of North America* 23(1), 25–40. DOI: 10.1016/j.chc.2013.08.001.

Gabriels, R.L., Pan, Z., Dechant, B., Agnew, J.A., Brim, N. et al. (2015) Randomized controlled trial of therapeutic horseback riding in children and adolescents with autism spectrum disorder. *Journal of the American Academy of Child and Adolescent Psychiatry* 54(7), 541–549. DOI: 10.1016/j.jaac.2015.04.007.

Grandin, T. (2019) Case study: how horses helped a teenager with autism make friends and learn how to work. *International Journal of Environmental Research and Public Health* 16(13), 2325. DOI: 10.3390/ijerph16132325.

Kaat, A.J., Lecavalier, L. and Aman, M.G. (2014) Validity of the aberrant behavior checklist in children with autism spectrum disorder. *Journal of Autism and Developmental Disorders* 44(5), 1103–1116. DOI: 10.1007/s10803-013-1970-0.

McDaniel Peters, B.C. and Wood, W. (2017) Autism and equine-assisted interventions: a systematic mapping review. *Journal of Autism and Developmental Disorders* 47(10), 3220–3242. DOI: 10.1007/s10803-017-3219-9.

Professional Association of Therapeutic Horsemanship, International (2020) Fact sheet 2020. Available at: https://pathintl.org/wp-content/uploads/2022/03/PATH-facts-2022.pdf (accessed 20 January 2023).

Stins, J.F. and Emck, C. (2018) Balance performance in autism: a brief overview. *Frontiers in Psychology* 9, 901. DOI: 10.3389/fpsyg.2018.00901.

Wood, W., Alm, K., Benjamin, J., Thomas, L., Anderson, D. et al. (2021) Optimal terminology for services in the United States that incorporate horses to benefit people: a consensus document. *Journal of Alternative and Complementary Medicine* 27(1), 88–95. DOI: 10.1089/acm.2020.0415.

9 Striking a Balance Between Welfare and Therapeutic Progress in Equine-assisted Services

MEGAN FRENCH* AND ANGELA FOURNIER

Eagle Vista Ranch, Bemidji, Minnesota, USA

Abstract

Equine-assisted services is a growing field in which horses are incorporated into interventions for human health and well-being. This chapter describes the different roles of mental health practitioners and equine specialists when incorporating horses in psychotherapy or learning sessions, particularly as it relates to welfare of the humans and horses involved. Welfare is primarily maintained by monitoring horse behavior and herd dynamics before and during sessions. We describe using ethograms to monitor horse maintenance behaviors and discuss welfare-process dilemmas, where welfare risks and therapeutic process are at odds. Case scenarios are provided, illustrating the balance between safety concerns and therapeutic benefit.

Our Background

We are a facilitation team, certified by the Equine Assisted Growth and Learning Association (Eagala). We use a ground-based approach where a mental health professional and an equine specialist work alongside one or more live horses on the ground (i.e. no horseback riding). We provide services at Eagle Vista Ranch & Wellness Center, a private practice in Northern Minnesota, co-facilitating both group and individual sessions, incorporating horses into psychotherapy and learning. Together, we work to create and hold a safe space for clients to engage with the horses and find solutions, offering support and helping them process their experience. Our individual roles call us to focus on specific aspects of welfare.

Client Welfare

I (Angela) am the mental health specialist on the facilitation team. I have a PhD in clinical psychology and am a licensed psychologist. I'm certified in equine-assisted intervention through both Eagala and the OK Corral Series. My role when co-facilitating equine sessions is to focus on the client, their goals for the session, and their behavior during the session as it relates to the treatment/intervention plan. My primary concerns during the session are the client's emotional safety and therapeutic progress.

Equine Welfare

I (Megan) am the equine specialist for our team. My training includes 5 years of experience with horses, working at a dressage barn and a pleasure horse farm. I have a bachelor's degree in psychology and am a certified equine specialist with Eagala. Regarding equine-assisted work, my role is to monitor the physical safety of the clients, horses, and facilitation team as well as noting shifts or patterns in the horses' behavior that may be relevant to the goals of the session. I make decisions to

*Corresponding author: mnfrench27@gmail.com

© CAB International 2024. *Animal-assisted Interventions: Recognizing and Mitigating Potential Welfare Challenges* (ed. L.R. Kogan)
DOI: 10.1079/9781800622616.0009

monitor and maintain welfare before and during the session.

Before the session

Well before the session, I start the process of selecting which horses will participate. This happens through monitoring the horses for any health conditions, injuries, or behavior inconducive to participating in a session. I watch for behavior from the horses suggesting they need a break from interacting with clients (e.g. atypical avoidance). If a horse has a physical limitation or injury, I limit the number of activities they participate in. In addition to determining which horses are sound to participate in a session, client preference is a factor. Returning clients may have a connection with a particular horse, and horses can become characters or symbols in the client's story.

During the session

Throughout the session, it is important that we as a facilitation team stand where we can see the whole herd and the client. I rely on my experience and training on natural horse behavior to assess risk and potential need for intervention. If there is conflict between horses that could be dangerous, I might separate them from one another or remove one from the session. Sometimes the client's behavior can create physical risk, if they scare a horse or aren't watching when horses are moving. Sessions sometimes include props (e.g. pool noodles, wooden blocks) for making paths or representations. The horses could be at risk if they chew on these props, or they can sometimes trip or spook from the props. In all of these situations, I am observing everyone's behavior, estimating risk, and preparing to intervene if needed. Intervening could mean saying something or moving in a way that shifts the client or horses out of the risky situation. Monitoring these large, notable behaviors is important to avoid acute welfare issues. As a team, we also measure moment-to-moment horse behavior across time to understand more long-term welfare factors.

Observing Maintenance Behavior

We use ethograms—lists of specific behaviors—to record basic maintenance behaviors (e.g. standing, moving, grazing) of each horse. We do this by scanning the pasture every 2 min for a sample of time. Doing this periodically allows us to observe and become familiar with each horse's typical behavior. This can be useful to monitor the horse's health, identifying changes in behavior (e.g. a horse grazing less than usual) that could indicate a health problem, an environmental hazard, or disruption in the herd. We make these same observations before, during, and after some equine sessions. This allows us to see how much the session is impacting or disrupting the horses' natural behavior. For example, if a horse typically grazes for 65% of the day but on session days only grazes 40% of the day, is their physical or mental health being affected? Ethograms can also be used to record human–horse behaviors like petting or grooming. Doing this has allowed us to see that while most of the herd experiences similar amounts of hands-on interaction with clients, one of our horses receives a lot more interaction and another receives a lot less. If we see signs of stress in the horses, we could explore whether it is related to the amount of human interaction and if so, find ways to reduce the workload.

Balancing Welfare and the Therapeutic Process

During equine sessions, we as a facilitation team work together to allow clients to engage with the horses in a meaningful way while monitoring the physical and emotional safety of the clients and horses. Some situations cause what we call a welfare-process dilemma, wherein there is a concern for the safety or well-being of the horses and/or humans involved, but intervening to reduce the risk could potentially interfere with the therapeutic process. In these situations, the facilitation team must grapple with whether to step in to reduce the risk, or to let the situation play out for possible therapeutic benefit. Thankfully, we are a team and can consult with each other right there, in the session. We assess the situation from each of our distinct roles—how is this relevant to the client's treatment goals and what are the potential consequences of interrupting the process happening (mental health specialist), and what are the risks to the horses and humans and the consequences of those risks (equine specialist). This cost–benefit analysis happens quickly. We decide together how to balance the certainty and severity of injury with the potential for therapeutic benefit. If deemed necessary, we intervene in the way that least disrupts the process. To most effectively resolve these dilemmas, we need to: (i) be familiar with the individual horses and the herd; (ii) communicate and trust each other as a team; and (iii) work within our roles as mental health and equine specialists. Below are two case scenarios illustrating welfare-process dilemmas.

Case Example I: Tower of Trouble

Employees from the local Department of Corrections were engaging in an equine-assisted learning session to address job stress and improve teamwork. After meeting the herd of eight horses, they decided to build something to represent their struggles on the job. They used materials in the arena to create a structure made of PVC pipes standing on end, leaning on each other, held together by a hula hoop, all surrounding a large barrel. The structure was standing quite tall and only loosely held together. The group came together around the tower and shared more about their challenges. They were listening to each other and making connections. In the meantime, several horses meandered into the space. One of the horses started to sniff the pipes and stuck his head between the pipes to sniff the barrel. While doing so, he was walking around the pipes barely missing them with his hooves. Just as the group's process was deepening the risk was escalating.

Discussion questions

1. What are the welfare risks in this scenario?
2. What would you do if you were the equine specialist?

Case Example II: Balance with Buckwheat

Our herd includes a miniature horse named Buckwheat, a 29-year-old gelding with a white coat, tail, and mane. He stands 8.5 hands tall and has lived and worked at the ranch for 7 years at the time of this writing. Buckwheat is *adorable*! His size, color, and conformation make him stand out in the herd. Clients notice him immediately and

often want to pet him. Buckwheat was rehomed to our ranch from previous owners and while much of his history is unknown, it is suspected he has experienced some trauma(s) in his life. He is intimidated by most horses and people, moving away whenever approached. He is quite difficult to catch and getting close enough to pet or groom him is a rarity. Still, he chooses to stay in proximity of the rest of the herd during sessions, rather than moving to another part of the pasture. The combination of his attractive physical appearance and avoidant response to virtually everyone sometimes creates a welfare-process dilemma. Clients approach him, wanting to interact with him and he moves away from them. Being avoided or rejected and struggling with trust are common issues addressed in psychotherapy. Failed attempts to engage Buckwheat can bring up a client's story around trust, belonging, and rejection. Working through those feelings, processing past events, and trying out new behaviors might be among the client's treatment goals. Working on these tasks by building trust with Buckwheat could be beneficial for the client but may be stressful for Buckwheat. Therein lies the welfare-process dilemma. Do we as facilitators allow the client to pursue Buckwheat and work on treatment goals but potentially cause him stress, or do we protect Buckwheat's well-being by asking the client not to pursue him and lose this opportunity for therapeutic change?

Discussion questions

1. What are the welfare concerns in this scenario?
2. What is the role of the equine specialist in making this decision?
3. What is the role of the mental health specialist in resolving this dilemma?

Acknowledgment

We are grateful to Liz Letson and the rest of the herd at Eagle Vista Ranch & Wellness Center for the experiences we've had that have informed this chapter.

10 Freedom, Choice, and Consent in the HERD

VERONICA LAC*

The HERD Institute, Orlando, Florida, USA

Abstract

This chapter introduces The HERD Institute® model of equine-facilitated work and highlights the importance of allowing for freedom, choice, and consent in both horses and humans in the relational process.

"The horses are in the arena waiting for you", said my host. As always, prior to partnering with any host facility, I had conducted a thorough facility assessment and emphasized the importance of a compassionate approach to working with horses from The HERD Institute® model of equine-facilitated work. We'd discussed the importance of giving our equine partners freedom and choice in how they engage with people during sessions, and the powerful impact for clients to witness consent in any interactions. So, I was a little surprised to discover that the horses were waiting for me in the indoor arena, tied to the walls with no hay or water. They didn't look distressed, uncomfortable, or agitated in any way, but I was curious why they had chosen to keep them tied up in the arena rather than at liberty in the adjoining outdoor paddock, and how long they had been waiting there. "They've only been there a couple of hours, but it's so that it's easier for us to catch them when we need them in whatever activity we do", said my host.

I smiled internally, bemused that I was being invited to present about my book *It's Not About the Activity: Thinking Outside the Toolbox in Equine Facilitated Psychotherapy and Learning* (Lac, 2020), only to be presented with this scenario at the start. I explained that if we needed to "catch" the horses, it would be a part of the process and that I would prefer to meet the horses in a more organic setting to see how they interact with me and with

each other rather than tied to the wall. This is part of the reason that I insist on spending time with the horses I'll be partnering with at any new facility. While I'll always request a staff member who knows the horses to be present throughout the day, I also need to have a sense of the herd dynamics, and quirks and characteristics of each horse, to maintain safety for both horses and humans. At The HERD Institute®, we subscribe to the idea that if it's not good for one, it's not good for all. Our methodology is based on a foundation of social justice, diversity, equity, and inclusion, and awareness of power, oppression, and cultural sensitivity issues are applied to both horses and humans, as they often emerge in the process in parallel. Rather than working with only metaphors, we attend to the actuality of the relationships that are formed in the moment.

The horses were released into the paddock. I spent some time with the herd, getting to know them in the presence of the two staff members, who were eager to tell me about their experiences of working with them. This workshop was designed for equine-facilitated practitioners who work with survivors of domestic abuse and/or sexual trafficking and the staff members were excited to be part of the group.

During the workshop, a theme emerged for the group centered on feelings of safety. When choice is available, even as experienced horse people,

---

*veronica@herdinstitute.com

there were differences in how safe each person felt in relation to horses they were unfamiliar with. The horses were turned loose in the arena and participants were invited to engage with them. A few people had chosen to groom the horses with brushes, a few had used their hands, and some had chosen to simply observe. I watched as one of the horses, who was being brushed by two women on either side of him, started to take a few steps forward. The women followed with a few steps forward. The horse stepped forward again. The women followed.

Me: I notice that Philippe took a few steps forward just now. What's happening for you both?

Annie: Oh, I didn't notice. I guess I just want to keep brushing him.

Mary: Me too. I noticed he moved but I was focusing on getting this bit of mud off him, I just carried on brushing.

Philippe took a few steps forward and turned, creating some space between him and the women, and positioned himself so that the women were now both on his left side.

Me: I see that Philippe moved again. What do you notice now?

Mary: I think he wants us to brush him on this side.

Annie: Maybe he didn't like being squashed in the middle? I guess it might feel a little claustrophobic with both of us brushing him at the same time.

Me: How are our themes of safety and choice showing up in this relationship with Philippe right now?

Mary: Well, I was so focused on doing something *to* him that I wasn't paying any attention to how he was reacting, so that's not very safe on my part. And I didn't ask him if it was OK to brush him, so I didn't offer him a choice. I suppose we could continue to brush him and see if he moves away from us again. If he does, I'd take that as him preferring not to have us touch him, and we can find a different way to connect?

Annie: Or we could take turns to brush him to see if it's about having too many people around him? I mean, he seems to be willing to stand with us right now.

This interaction provided a nuanced example of how to work relationally with the horses and led to a discussion on how safety and choice is only possible when we intentionally look for feedback from others. One participant commented that this was particularly relevant for them in working with survivors of domestic violence and/or sexual trafficking, and that even the act of following Philippe step by step, could potentially be reminiscent of the micro-level of control that their clients may have experienced. Another participant highlighted that just because Philippe seemed calm and not highly activated (e.g. running away), it didn't mean that he was necessarily consenting to being brushed, and that there's a difference between consent and compliance, again, something that their client population would resonate with.

This theme resurfaced later when the group chose to work with just one of the horses in the adjoining pasture. Katie led the chestnut mare, Amber, into the pasture and took off her halter. Amber stood in the center, lifted her head, stretched out her neck and sniffed the air, before slowly walking to the fence line separating her from the other horses. Katie had exited the pasture to rejoin the rest of the group outside. I had checked with a staff member about whether separating Amber from the herd would cause any anxiety and had been assured that she would be fine. So, I was surprised when Amber suddenly took off, running the length of the pasture along the fence line, tail in the air, whinnying as she went. The rest of the herd were on the far side of the adjoining pasture. A couple of them lifted their heads, but most of them carried on grazing. We watched as Amber became increasingly agitated, pawing at the ground and the wooden fence. I knew that in that moment, my choices were to ask the participants to share their perspectives of what was happening while allowing Amber to continue expressing herself, or to intervene in some way to help Amber to regulate. While I recognized that the first option could provide insights for the participants, I did not want to sacrifice Amber's well-being for that purpose.

"I see that Amber is getting activated right now, so for her well-being, I'm going to ask Katie to go and halter her and we'll lead her back to the other side. While we do that, I invite you all to notice how Amber is responding to Katie's presence and what you're feeling as you witness all this," I said. Katie walked up to Amber slowly, calling her name gently, letting out a deep exhale as she approached.

The mare turned and exhaled. Katie continued to breathe deeply as she reached up to put the halter on and slowly led Amber back towards the rest of the herd. Once she was back in the adjoining pasture, Amber stayed by the fence line where the participants had gathered. I asked the group what they were experiencing in that moment.

Katie: I feel better now that she's more settled. I didn't like seeing her so distressed just now, so I'm glad you asked me to bring her back in here.

Annie: Yes, me too. I had this story in my head that she felt like no one cared when she was in distress because none of the other horses came over to check on her when she was calling out to them.

Rachel: I felt myself settling as Katie approached her. I didn't realize that I was so tense watching Amber getting activated.

Tony: At the risk of upsetting everyone, I think she would've been fine after a few minutes. I'm not sure it was necessary to move her back. Sometimes they need to learn to self-regulate. I mean, it's not like you were asking very much of her, and she wasn't really "working".

Discussion Questions

1. What would you have done in this situation with Amber?
2. What do you do (or would you do) when your equine partner(s) show distress?
3. What do you define as "working" for your horses?
4. How often do you find yourself saying "I'm not asking much of you" to your equine partners? What impact might this have?
5. How might this scenario translate into human interactions, specifically for the client population that this group works with?
6. What power dynamics are at play that may parallel client experiences?

Since this workshop was aimed at equine-facilitated practitioners working with survivors of domestic violence and/or sexual trafficking, the themes that emerged allowed group members to recognize the importance of allowing for freedom and choice for their equine partners in the work. The direct parallels that these clients can draw from witnessing how we treat our horses in sessions with their lived experiences of being controlled, abused, abandoned, and feelings of powerlessness can be profound. Providing space for participants to interact with the horses from a place of freedom, choice, and consent allows them to begin to heal these wounds. Particularly, the expectation that because we feed and take care of our horses, we are entitled to ask them to "work" can lead to profound parallels for this client population.

Maya Angelou's oft quoted "Do the best you can until you know better. Then when you know better, do better" (Quote Investigator®, 2022) is something I hold closely in my relationship with horses. My own journey of being with horses, started from a dominance-based, hierarchical, power-over, human-centric approach. As I learned more about equine ethology, behavior, stress and pain signals, and a more compassionate way of being with them, I recognize that there is still so much that we don't know about these magnificent animals. I'm careful about the language that we use when talking about incorporating horses into any learning or psychotherapy intervention, because it matters to me that what I say and what I do is aligned; that the philosophy, theory, and practice of equine-facilitated interventions that we teach are consistent. If we claim to be in awe of the wisdom of horses, and believe in their sentience, we need to be mindful of how we can so easily "do to" rather than "be with" them. We need to acknowledge the difference between compliance and consent, pay attention to the non-verbal communication of our animal partners, and be clear that they are not tools to be used, but equal partners in the process.

References

Lac, V. (2020) *It's Not About the Activity: Thinking Outside the Toolbox of Equine Facilitated Psychotherapy and Learning*. University Professors Press, Colorado Springs, Colorado.

Quote Investigator® (2022). Available at: https://quoteinvestigator.com/2022/11/30/did-better/ (accessed 2 March 2023).

11 Acknowledging and Mitigating Professional Compassion Fatigue: Personal Reflections on Animal-assisted Work

ELIZABETH A. LETSON[1,2]* AND JOY R. HANSON[3]

[1]Owner and CEO, Eagle Vista Ranch & Wellness Center, Bemidji, Minnesota, USA; [2]Bemidji State University, Bemidji, Minnesota, USA; [3]Colorado Christian University, Lakewood, Colorado, USA

Abstract

For helping professionals—whether they work with animals, people, or both—compassion fatigue is a significant and enduring obstacle to helping others and to maintaining personal wellness, ethical imperatives for counselors and other helping professionals. With the overarching goal of raising awareness of compassion fatigue as a welfare issue, its antecedents, and how it can be mitigated, this chapter examines one of the author's personal experiences with compassion fatigue, burnout, and building resilience. The authors also describe research-based methods of mitigating compassion fatigue and point to the necessity of practitioners building resilience and finding sustaining personal and professional passions.

Working in the mental health field, and animal-assisted intervention (AAI) work in particular, poses a unique set of welfare challenges, including managing both two-legged and four-legged chronic health conditions, facing difficult end-of-life decisions for horses and other animals, and the ramifications of those conditions and decisions on clients and the rest of the two- and four-legged team. Additionally, mental health practices utilizing AAI are not immune to ordinary professional and personal challenges. For over 11 years, I (Liz) have owned and worked in a private equine- and animal-assisted practice as a licensed professional clinical counselor and have come to know firsthand the welfare challenges faced by both practitioners and clients. A personal hurdle in my mental health practice is compassion fatigue, a common challenge among professionals in all the caring fields. Compassion fatigue, used to describe

the physical, emotional, and psychological impact of caring for others—particularly those who have experienced trauma—can lead to burnout if not actively mitigated. In my own work as an equine-assisted private practice owner and practitioner, I have experienced AAI as a very effective personal and professional mitigation strategy in the treatment and support of compassion fatigue. But, in this chapter, I share my *personal* experience with compassion fatigue, the tools I use to work through it, and how it has catapulted me into the next "chapter" of my professional life.

The year 2022 was a tumultuous one. I was still reeling from the effects of the coronavirus disease 2019 (COVID-19) pandemic on my private practice, including having to rehome three of my therapy horses, who are my four-legged family. My two-legged family members were also having some issues of their own which were far-reaching

*Corresponding author: eaglevistaranch@gmail.com

© CAB International 2024. *Animal-assisted Interventions: Recognizing and Mitigating Potential Welfare Challenges* (ed. L.R. Kogan)
DOI: 10.1079/9781800622616.0011

and consumed much of my time and energy. My own physical health was also an issue. First, one of my horses, Crackerjack, who had been with me since 2001, passed away suddenly and unexpectedly. Much like losing a beloved family member, I felt great anger and grief at the loss. That I was not present when he died led to feelings of guilt, as well. Even more heartbreaking to me was what transpired with two of my other therapy horses. I knew the mare and gelding siblings, Montana and Dakota, who had come to my practice in 2014, would not survive another harsh Minnesota winter, due to deteriorating health and advanced age (both were in their upper 30s). After consultation with the ranch veterinarian, I had to make a painful, but necessary decision—a decision I did not take lightly—to have them euthanized. As if to add insult to injury, I was also dealing with back and hip pain following an uncharacteristic outburst from another of my therapy horses, Superman, a senior off-the-track thoroughbred who has been with me since 2007. He kicked me in the butt! (Talk about a metaphor.)

While animal-assisted work is immensely rewarding, it can also be incredibly challenging, as my own experiences illustrate. Ethically speaking, all individuals in the helping professions must care for themselves (Skovholt and Trotter-Mathison, 2016), ensuring they are mentally, emotionally, and physically up to the task of caring for and helping others. In AAI, however, practitioners must also consider the welfare of the animals with whom they partner, ensuring the horses and other animals are mentally, emotionally, and physically fit for the work. AAI professionals face a number of pain points, or aspects of the profession which are uniquely challenging or emotionally depleting. In my own work, I have faced the pain points of equine health issues, particularly end-of-life decisions, injuries, and the balancing of my needs and those of my clients with the horses' needs and welfare. The needs of my two-legged team members, including interns and other colleagues, must also be considered. These pain points, as well as many difficulties and stressors in my health and personal life, left me feeling fatigued, emotionally exhausted, frustrated, depleted, and even questioning aspects of my life and work. These struggles I was experiencing were no longer isolated to the work I was doing, but touched the deepest parts of myself. I realized I was deep in compassion fatigue and well on my way to burnout.

What does a seasoned mental health professional do when she realizes she is suffering from compassion fatigue? In my case, the losses in both my two- and four-legged families had me working through the emotional processes of Dr. Kübler-Ross's (1969) stages of grief: denial, anger, bargaining, depression, and acceptance, often referred to as the DABDA model. While there are other grief models in use, this is a popular model for understanding the stages of grief, and its familiar language was a source of comfort in my mourning.

In the midst of all this tumult, I realized I had to take my own advice and "feel it to heal it". I could not walk away from the grief, anger, guilt, and frustration, but needed to firmly plant my two feet and "feel the feels", as one of my clients says about his own journey (I often find wisdom in what clients have to say). Reducing my workload gave me the emotional and intellectual space to process my grief and talk to my two-legged team. It also allowed me the time to talk with my veterinarian and farrier who both helped me to process through the stages of grief. Walking my dogs, Bronco and Moose, and hanging out with my herd in the pasture became my own form of AAI. Managing compassion fatigue and burnout is never a linear process, it's more like a winding road, and one I'm still traveling. Along with seeking the comfort of my two- and four-legged team members, and friends and family, I also sought out mental health therapy for myself, which gave me not only hope and healing, but the opportunity to experience what it felt like to be on the other side of the compassion fatigue dynamic.

As I became more intentional about my self-care and priorities, reducing my workload, and processing how these experiences had impacted me emotionally and intellectually, I felt old passions reignited. I resumed playing the piano, singing, and skiing. Several years ago, I started work focusing on resilience in the helping professions and was greatly inspired by Skovholt and Trotter-Mathison's (2016) book, *The Resilient Practitioner: Burnout and Compassion Fatigue Prevention and Self-Care Strategies for the Helping Professions*, which offers resources and strategies for managing compassion fatigue, particularly for those in the helping professions. For Skovholt and Trotter-Mathison, the solution to compassion fatigue and other challenges, which they term hazards of practice, is resilience. Put simply, resilience is the ability to bounce back, especially from stressful situations. In addition to ordinary self-care, the authors identify several other key strategies to build resilience and help practitioners sustain their professional selves. These include: (i) choosing meaningful work; (ii) relishing small victories; (iii) thinking long-term; (iv) intentionally and actively engaging in self-development; and (v) working towards professional self-understanding. The authors also emphasize the importance of caring for the personal self, in all its facets, including the emotional, loving, physical, recreational, and spiritual selves, among many others. Striving for self-awareness, working towards emotional well-being, and prioritizing mutually supportive personal relationships are also crucial to the practitioner's long-term personal and professional survival and resilience.

Many of the strategies I was using in my own life to become more resilient mirrored those outlined by Skovholt and Trotter-Mathison (2016). When I realized this, I was energized to share the knowledge and tools with others in the helping professions, to help them avoid compassion fatigue and become more resilient. This insight has spurred me to network with AAI practitioners in other states, promoting an outreach program utilizing equine-assisted learning (EAL) for animal care staff, healers, caregivers, and helping professionals in self-care and resiliency. Most affirming and exciting for me is my renewed interest in building an online curriculum that is resilience based, addressing the pain points that AAI practitioners experience. Offering language to describe what practitioners experience, as well as providing understanding and awareness that we are not alone on this journey are so important. My hope for this resiliency program is that it will provide actionable steps to lead individuals from exhaustion and fatigue to a place where a community of AAI folks can offer ideas, strategies, and hope—a community where we can share, learn, and grow. The best lessons, it seems, come from life itself and from sharing the lessons of our lives with others.

I wish I had known about compassion fatigue, burnout, and the various hazards of practice when I first began graduate school. Since then, in my work as a counselor and in AAI, I have struggled with having excessive empathy for people and for animals, and did not realize how much I was pushing myself to the point of burnout. Through a deeper understanding of compassion fatigue, as well as the help of my two- and four-legged team members, my own resilience and my passion for helping other professionals along their resilience journeys has been reignited. This chapter is dedicated to other practitioners who, like me, struggle to mitigate their own personal compassion fatigue. It chronicles my own journey through compassion fatigue with a tour through burnout alley, links my own experiences to important research in the field of resilience, and describes how these experiences have catapulted me into the next chapter of helping other practitioners rise into their own resilience, allowing them to serve others without depleting themselves. My co-author is a counseling student who is relatively new to the field and has already benefited greatly from understanding the dynamics of compassion fatigue, burnout, and resilience from early in her career. In sharing my story with her, I grew to appreciate more deeply the need for helping professionals to implement these strategies early and consistently throughout their own careers. I hope our own experiences can encourage other practitioners and inspire them to build their own resilience, increase their personal and professional vitality, and to pursue their passions.

Discussion Questions

1. In your own life, how have you experienced compassion fatigue and burnout? How have you worked to mitigate these challenges?
2. How have you utilized self-care, coping strategies, and other resources to build your resilience? What strategies have been helpful or unhelpful? What strategies would you share with other AAI professionals?

References

Kübler-Ross, E. (1969) *On Death and Dying: What the Dying Have to Teach Doctors, Nurses, Clergy and their own Families*. MacMillan, London.
Skovholt, T.M. and Trotter-Mathison, M. (2016) *The Resilient Practitioner: Burnout and Compassion Fatigue Prevention and Self-Care Strategies for the Helping Professions*, 3rd edn. Routledge, New York. DOI: 10.4324/9781315737447.

12 Time to Say Goodbye: Honoring the Life and Death of a Therapy Horse

ARIEAHN MATAMONASA-BENNETT*

Licensed Psychologist and equine-assisted psychotherapy (EAP) practitioner, Chicago, Illinois, USA

Abstract

There is a paucity of literature on the dying and grief process of people and their companion animals, and even less on the therapy animals who partner with practitioners in animal-assisted therapies (AATs). Given the intimate and deeply meaningful relationships both practitioners and their clients form with the therapy animals they work with, this deserves more in-depth examination. This is true for the human clients and therapists, as well as for the animals themselves. In the practice of equine-assisted therapy (EAT) the horse is not a tool or a metaphor, but rather a sentient being with a subjective self and partner to the therapists they work with.

Almost a decade ago, I researched and published a study on ethical issues in equine-assisted therapy (EAT) relationships that included how end of life and other difficult decisions about the health and welfare of horses were considered by over 100 EAT practitioners (Matamonasa-Bennett, 2015). What I found most surprising is that many of the practitioners had not considered these issues in a formal way, but seemed to handle things on a case-by-case individual-situation basis. When the call for chapters came for this volume, I knew immediately that I had a story to tell. The goal here is not to be prescriptive, as I have in other writings, but rather give the reader something to consider about these issues from the lens of my lived experience.

Savannah

Savannah was a rescue horse who had been abandoned by her owners at the lesson barn that hosted my EAT practice and was "free to a good home"—headed to what we in the horse world call "the cheap auction" or the slaughter pen. She was in her mid-teens and other than being out of physical shape and badly needing her feet and teeth done, was otherwise healthy. In a tack trunk that came with the horse I found a journal from years before when the owners purchased her as a child's Christmas gift and it was clear from the entries that the original enthusiasm was quickly curbed by the stark reality of the time, effort, energy, and expense of caring for her. Sadly, this is not a rare situation.

She was a quiet mare (mostly), but also sensitive to people and needed to become reoriented to grooming, handling, and attention. After several months of working with her, I decided to try her in my therapy program. She turned out to be an amazing therapy horse and I learned much from working with her. We developed a strong bond and worked with hundreds of clients over the next decade. Many early articles and research I did featured the work we did in our partnership (Matamonasa-Bennett, 2010, 2011). In 2014, she fell ill and was diagnosed with Cushing's disease.[1] We managed this with medications, special dietary changes, and continued lots of turnout and social time until 2017 when her symptoms worsened and the medications and management were becoming less effective.

*amatamo1@depaul.edu

DOI: 10.1079/9781800622616.0012

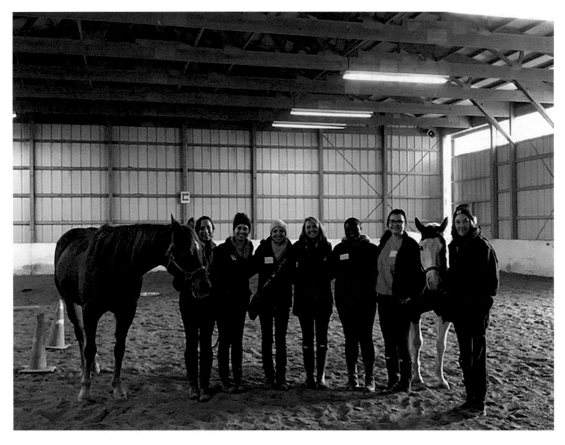

Fig. 12.1. Savannah's last therapy session with a college group, October, 2017.

Freedom of choice

I have written about and practiced the importance of freedom of choice for horses doing EAT and starting in the fall of that year, Savannah indicated on several occasions through specific behaviors (i.e. earpinning, turning away) that she did not want to engage with clients in therapy sessions. Other times she seemed eager to join the sessions and connect with clients. I had other horses that I could work with—so this was not an issue in my practice although I greatly missed having my reliable partner with whom I had developed such a close bond and working relationship. My other horses were very good but Savannah was extraordinary. On October 28, 2017, I hosted a college class for an all-day experiential workshop on EAT and this was Savannah's last session (Fig. 12.1). I was attuned and attentive enough to her to know that she was done with doing this work.

Giving clients a chance to say goodbye

I decided to officially retire Savannah from being a therapy horse and I also wanted to make sure that I could give our clients, both present and past, an opportunity to say goodbye and to visit her and tell her how much she meant to them. I chose the following weekend and hosted an open house when clients could come during open-barn hours to visit her. The response was overwhelming. The adults who had worked with her over the last 10 years came, kids who were now in college came back, and current families came and brought notes and cards that they hung on her stall (Fig. 12.2). While I have a practice of always making sure clients thank my horses at the end of each session, I really believe that with these visits she could feel and understand how loved and appreciated she was by these clients.

My plan was to let her live out her days with the highest quality, keeping her as comfortable and

A. Matamonasa-Bennett

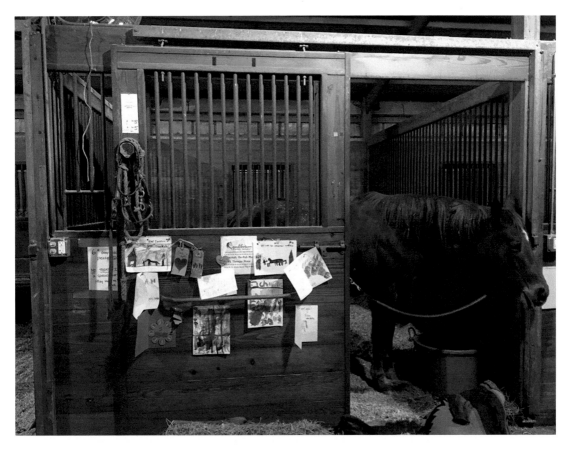

Fig. 12.2. Savannah's stall with cards from clients at the open house for her retirement.

painfree as possible. When her condition worsened and I could not manage her pain I began to discuss euthanasia with my vet. This was agonizing—but when she stopped eating and refused to come out of her stall to go outside, I knew that the time had come to let her go and to be courageous enough to see her through this process in a sacred way.

Creating a ceremonial space to honor her life

As a cross-culturally trained psychologist from a depth orientation (exploring the unconscious thought using seemingly insignificant events such as slips of the tongue, spontaneous humor, dreams, and coincidences), creating rituals for individuals and groups was a natural practice for me. I even conceptualized EAT sessions as a form of ritual. For example, the check in or preparation for the session typically took place outside the horse arena, and once we entered the arena with the horses

this became a sacred, non-ordinary space where the healing and learning could occur. Like rituals, the sessions had a beginning, middle, climax, end and summary for integration of the work into the ordinary, everyday world. Beyond EAT sessions, I had created many rituals for helping individuals and groups with psychological and spiritual transitions—including death. I was often called upon to create rituals and assist with humans as their companion animals or horses transitioned. I naturally wanted to create a ritual for Savannah but doing this in the midst of my own grief was more difficult than I imagined.

I scheduled the vet to come on the Wednesday before Thanksgiving. The barn was sure to be very quiet that day. I asked my daughter and a few close friends and my long-time farrier to be there to assist with creating a sacred way to let her transition. This horse who partnered in so much human healing deserved a spiritual honoring at the end of her life. I decided to have everyone write tiny prayers for her transition to put into a cloth bundle that I then tied with a ribbon to her mane. I brushed her and braided her tail. My daughter burned sage and we all formed a circle around her and each person approached her and said their prayers and goodbyes. I thanked Savannah out loud for everything she had done for me and all the people she had worked with. There was not a dry eye in that circle, including the vet and the farrier who is a tough-as-nails, rodeo cowboy. When she was gone, I covered her with a blanket and cut off her tail to keep and I waited for the cremation service to come. I took the next 5 days off from my practice. My dreams those nights were filled with Savannah, almost like watching her life in review.

I continue to love this work with my newer horses but it has never been the same without her. It has been 6 years now and this is the first time I have written about this. While the grief was deep

for me and for some of my clients, I believe that both the open house, providing the opportunity to say goodbye, as well as the end-of-life ritual that I created eased some of the loss and grief for me and those who knew her. I hoped that it models a way in which we can intentionally honor the healing contribution that horses make to our lives.

Bringing Savannah home

When Savannah was alive, I often talked to her about my dream to own my own farm with beautiful grass pastures. Ironically once she was diagnosed with Cushing's disease she would not have been able to enjoy *eating* the grass, but nonetheless I always daydreamed with her. I often promised her I was working on this dream and that we would have our own place one day. During the pandemic I found myself working exclusively remotely and this allowed me to move further from the city to

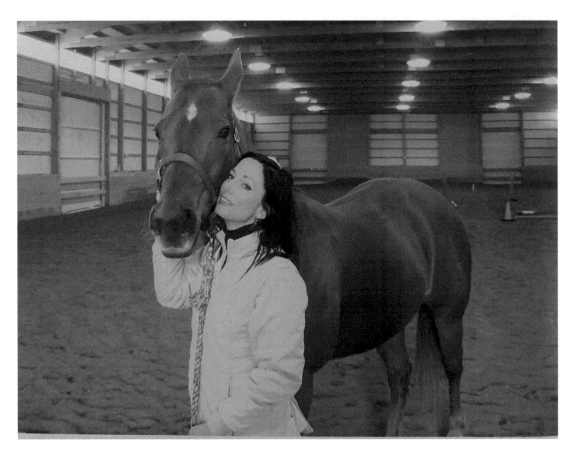

Fig. 12.3. Savannah in her prime with the author.

a more affordable region for horses. I bought my lifelong-dream horse property in the new year of 2021. In November of 2021, on the fourth anniversary of her passing, I sprinkled her ashes in my large pasture. Savannah is part of my home, my work and my continued relationship with horses. She still comes into my dreams and my journey-work (Fig. 12.3).

I have on my left shoulder, a replica of a tattoo from the Bronze Age Pazyryk culture who are believed to be the first equestrians. My dear friend and scholar Gala Argent studied these tattoos and published her theory that the tattoos represented all the horses in a person's life, as bonds with horses were central to everything in their culture. The tattoos were symbolic representations of the "babysitter" (horse) who taught the person to ride as a child, the horse of the person's mid-life and the horse of a lifetime (Argent, 2013). I did keep a small amount of Savannah's ashes which I will mix in the ink of my next tattoo—*but that* will be for another chapter.

Discussion Questions

1. What might be some reasons many practitioners of animal-assisted therapy (AAT) do not formally think about or plan for end-of-life issues for the animals they work with?

2. What things might complicate the grief process surrounding a therapy animal when compared to a pet?

Note

[1] Cushing's disease in horses is also called pituitary pars intermedia dysfunction (PPID). It is a progressive neurodegenerative disorder in horses.

References

Argent, G. (2013) Inked: human-horse apprenticeship, tattoos, and time in the Pazyryk world. *Society and Animals* 21(2), 178–193. DOI: 10.1163/15685306-12341301.

Matamonasa-Bennett, A. (2010) Case studies show merit for equine assisted psychotherapy research. *Human Animal Interaction Newsletter,* Human Animal Interaction Section (Published by the American Psychological Association).

Matamonasa-Bennett, A. (2011) Reading horses, reading people: improving social skills and awareness through equine assisted therapy. *Human Animal Interaction Newsletter,* Human Animal Interaction Section (Published by the American Psychological Association).

Matamonasa-Bennett, A. (2015) Putting the horse before Descartes: native American paradigms and ethics in equine assisted therapies. *Business and Professional Ethics Journal* 33(4), 23–43. DOI: 10.5840/bpej201562624.

13 Animal-assisted Interventions and the Lessons Learned—Striving for Safe, Sane, and Humane Interactions

Susan D. Greenbaum*

RxCanines – Therapeutic Intervention Dogs, Milford, New Jersey, USA

Abstract

The animal-assisted intervention (AAI) response to the events of September 11, 2001, at the Family Assistance Center at Liberty State Park in New Jersey had many welfare challenges. While 9/11 was a unique situation, there are lessons to be learned for all types of AAI work. Incorporating "Is it Safe? Is it Sane? Is it Humane?" helps set priorities for decisions in any situation.

The trauma therapist nodded to the dog–handler team and they all walked outside. The boy, who was 5 years old, slowly looked up. Then he looked down at the miniature pinscher. He stretched one hand up, as far as he could reach with the palm facing the ground. With the other, he reached as low as he could with the palm facing up. "Winnie, the building was this big" and then he brought his palms together "and now it is this big". There was a long pause. "I don't think mommy is coming home." Winnie, her handler, the therapist, and the boy stayed silent looking across the Hudson River at the smoldering pile at Ground Zero (Fig. 13.1).

The events of September 11, 2001, (hereafter 9/11) created a unique situation in the field of animal-assisted interventions (AAI), for example: (i) collaboration of different AAI organizations; (ii) having dogs and their handlers work in an unfamiliar environment; (iii) working more frequently for longer periods of time than usual for the team; and (iv) some traveling a much greater distance than was usual. These unusual conditions contribute to our understanding of animal welfare challenges during AAIs.

Security at the Family Assistance Center (FAC), one of two facilities set up near the catastrophe, was tight. When the program started, the AAI-overseeing organization, New Jersey (NJ) Department of Health and Human Services, Division of Mental Health, warned me we could be there for 4 weeks. It turned out to be closer to 5 months. Phases of the family assistance program included filing missing person reports, DNA gathering (where the families would be asked to bring a toothbrush, hairbrush or other item from the "missing" individual), issuing of death certificates, and the presentation of flags and urns. Through all phases, families were offered various assistance from housing subsidies to mental health services.

On the NJ side of the river, I was honored to be the AAI coordinator at Liberty State Park which housed the NJ FAC. Five animal-assisted activities (AAA)/animal-assisted therapies (AAT) organizations shared responsibility for covering the FAC

*Barkinghills@gmail.com

© CAB International 2024. *Animal-assisted Interventions: Recognizing and Mitigating Potential Welfare Challenges* (ed. L.R. Kogan)
DOI: 10.1079/9781800622616.0013

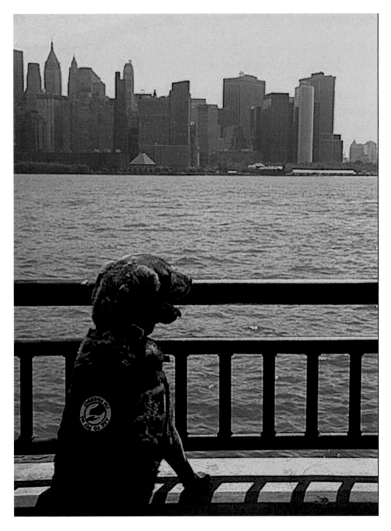

Fig. 13.1. Dog looking across the Hudson River.

from September of 2001 to the middle of January 2002. Teams worked with survivors, family members, relief workers, and first responders. When making decisions, often with little information and less time, the mantra of try and make it "Safe, Sane, and Humane" were our guiding principles:

- **Safe:** Safety of the dog, the handler, clients, and the public are paramount to the work.
- **Sane:** Sane interactions are possible with realistic expectations. These include the frequency and length of interactions, the number of clients being serviced, and the environment.
- **Humane:** Humane interactions can occur when the animal:
  - has the ability to give and withdraw consent;
  - is monitored for canine stress;
  - has work–life balance;
  - is physically fit;
  - is an appropriate age; and
  - is supervised by someone with the education and insight to monitor the interactions.

My Chesapeake Bay retriever and I were one of the 147 dog–handler teams on the NJ side, for 4.5 months at the FAC, while continuing our usual work at a children's hospital. Choosing which teams from my organization would work at the FAC and what working conditions would be used by all dog–handler teams was difficult, to put it mildly. Everyone wanted to help but all teams were not suited to do the work. That was difficult for some handlers to accept.

In NJ, organizations decided which of their members would be scheduled to work, how many hours (a maximum of 4 hours a day), and how many days of the week a team could work (a maximum of 3 days a week).

Considerations for scheduling decisions included:

- Team experience.
- Handler resilience.
- In which environments are they accustomed to working?
- What is the team's usual population? Adults? Geriatric? Pediatric? Psychiatric?
- Physical condition of the dog.
- Will the dog be comfortable in *this* environment?
- How far will the team travel?
- Daily temperature—it ranged from 30°F to 90°F (−1°C to 32°C) during the program. Some breeds, like brachycephalic breeds, are difficult to keep cool on a warm day. It is easier to warm a dog up than cool a dog down.

In October, ferries started running from the FACs to Ground Zero where families could see the site, and leave something in memory of their loved one. Children were provided with teddy bears they could leave or keep. As you can imagine, these were very emotional events.

The decision was made to send one dog–handler team per boat. As the NJ-based lead, I made the very unpopular decision to not cover the ferries coming from the NJ FAC. I was fortunate that I was given the authority to make this type of decision; others were not given the same autonomy. I believed the conditions, set by the ferries and state officials, to limit each ferry to one dog–handler team for 300+ extremely emotional people, with no quiet area for the team to go for a break, and the length of time of the trip (2+ hours) would not be a safe or sane working environment. It was an extremely difficult decision as we all wanted to do everything possible for the families. However, animal welfare and safety concerns were prioritized in the final

decision. From this experience I learned that sometimes acting as an advocate for the animals can be quite challenging and takes a great deal of strength and willingness to be the bad guy.

Of course, things don't always go according to plan. Normal coverage was three sets of teams, each working a 4-hour shift covering 12 hours a day. The ratio of people to teams was, at maximum, 50:1. Many people did not interact with the teams. One day I received a call from the head of an AAA organization who was extremely upset. Instead of the small group of relief workers I had told her to anticipate, there were close to 3000 grieving family members. The teams were overwhelmed and she was out for my head! Understandably. For security reasons, I had not been informed the families were returning back to the FAC after the distribution of American flags and urns containing remains. Had I known, we would have sent ten times the number of teams, in multiple shifts, or canceled the teams for that day. We joke about that phone call now but, at the time, it was a tense reminder of the limits of our daily information and constant need to adapt.

In 2003, after the FAC and our program shut down, one regional service-dog organization sent a survey to over 500 handlers who worked in NJ, New York, and Virginia. The survey covered many aspects of the 9/11 AAI response including: (i) how long the team worked; (ii) where they worked; (iii) how many times a week; (iv) length of the shifts; and (v) how far they traveled. Also it asked handlers about canine stressors, and whether or not they had returned to the AAI work they did prior to 9/11. There were almost 300 responses.

Perhaps the most telling lesson from the survey was the disconnect between handlers reporting of canine stress indicators and the canine burnout that occurred. Handlers denied observing canine stress signals from their partners but also reported their canine teammates had not returned to their previous work. Some were honest enough to report signs of aggression, to both canines and humans, in their previously reliable partner. It fascinated and disturbed me and spurred my interest in canine burnout.

As reported in the survey, things that impacted canine stress included:

- *Ability to rest undisturbed*—Dogs who were comfortable resting in a crate appeared to get a better quality of rest during down times and, as there was a physical barrier, people (including the handler) tended to leave the dogs alone to rest.

- *Ability to urinate and defecate on unfamiliar surfaces*—In New York City concrete was the norm and many dogs found it difficult to find a place to "go".
- *Comfort traveling*—Carpooling meant traveling in an unfamiliar car with other dogs who may, or may not, be familiar.
- *Length of time working and numbers of days per week worked*—The closer to the dogs' usual routine, the fewer stress indicators reported.
- *Handler stress*—Dogs with stressed handlers, whether from outside factors or the work itself, were more stressed.
- *Crowd control*—Maintaining the dog's "personal space" was important to avoid keeping the dog from feeling surrounded or trapped (i.e. one person, one hand at a time, avoided hugs which many dogs found uncomfortable).
- *Ability of the team to self-monitor*—The temptation to work "five more minutes" or fill in because there are not enough teams is one familiar to anyone who does AAI work and can lead to canine burnout. I know I came quite close to burning out my own dog post-9/11.

An important factor was canine consent. Our canine partners need to be willing and active participants. Consent is given in each working moment. This includes the dog: (i) putting on working gear (as opposed to the gear being put on the dog); (ii) eagerly loading into a car or other mode of transportation; and (iii) happily engaging with people when permitted. Consent is contextual: a dog may consent with one individual and not another, consent at one time and not another, on one day and not another. A dog may consent to be touched on the back but not the top of the head, and so on.

Consent is critical in AAI:

- A dog who is able to decide when to engage/disengage is less likely to experience high levels of stress.

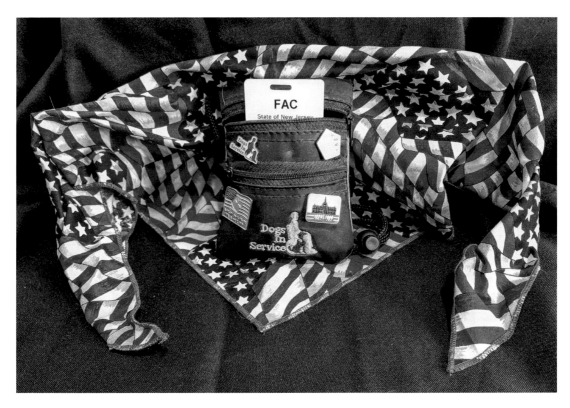

Fig. 13.2. Dog bandana and Family Assistance Center (FAC) ID.

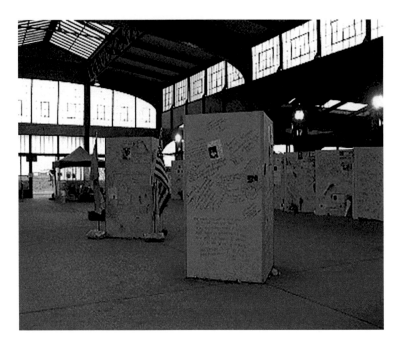

Fig. 13.3. FAC memory walls.

- Dogs who work on a tight lead, are held, or are confined to a stroller or carrier, lack the ability to approach or retreat and therefore cannot consent.
- Similarly, a dog who is responding to a cue (i.e. "Say Hello") lacks the ability to consent.

Dogs who are bred to work separately from people (hounds, Nordic breeds, terriers, etc.) intrinsically show greater ability to give and withdraw consent. When a dog is bred to work with people (think retrievers, herding breeds, mixes of these, and similar dogs), *and* a dog is well trained, *and* is well bonded with the handler, there is greater risk of burnout. These dogs will do whatever we ask of them regardless of their own desires. Long term, however, they are likely to pay the price.

It's dark and some police officers are hanging out, looking across
the Hudson at "the pile". My dog's
flag bandana falls off (Fig. 13.2).
An officer kneels and ties it back
on my dog before I can intervene. I
hear him whisper softly to the dog:
"What's the matter buddy? Are you sad

because there isn't anyone here you
can help?"

We all wanted to help. Our desire to incorporate our canine partners was well intentioned. But we learned from the experience at the FAC (Fig. 13.3) that our desire to help needs to be tempered by "Safe, Sane, and Humane". We owe it to our working partners to prioritize consent and minimize factors leading to burnout. It certainly isn't easy. And not always popular! Making decisions based on whether something is safe, sane, and humane is challenging, but it is one of the best ways to preserve the working life of the dog. It is what having true partnership with our dogs is about.

Discussion Questions

1. What types of handler education are needed for "Safe, Sane, and Humane" interactions?
2. What does allowing the dog to give and withdraw consent to go to work, when to start or finish an interaction, etc., add to "Safe, Sane, and Humane" working conditions?

S.D. Greenbaum

14 Animal-assisted Crisis Response: The Balance Between Work and Welfare

BATYA G. JAFFE*

Wurzweiler School of Social Work, Yeshiva University, New York, USA

Abstract

This chapter discusses the handler's responsibilities to their dog while working to help survivors of crises and disasters. Animal-Assisted Crisis Response (AACR) is an innovative tool that helps survivors who have undergone trauma. To ensure an effective application of this intervention, handlers must learn how to prioritize and secure the welfare and safety of their dogs.

Introduction

The Psychotrauma Unit in Israel is a unit within the United Hatzalah of Israel (a non-profit organization that attends medical emergencies) that responds to crises and disasters intending to stabilize trauma survivors. Survivors, bystanders, and family members may suffer from mental, as well as physical, harm as a result of experiencing a natural disaster or crisis situation. Stabilizing and comforting trauma survivors can change how they respond to the trauma and speed up their journey toward healing. A unique way to help trauma survivors is through Animal-Assisted Crisis Response (AACR).

After joining the Psychotrauma Unit in Israel, I understood the advantages of working with canines—for me, this entails working with Lucy, my wonderful Cavalier King Charles Spaniel.

While living in Israel, whenever an ambulance was deployed, I was called, together with Lucy, to assess and treat survivors of tragedies ranging from sudden infant death syndrome (SIDS) and suicides to terrorist attacks, building collisions, and more. The lessons I learned and the experience I gained throughout my career in the field helped guide my future practice and research. These experiences also motivated me to broaden my horizon and collaborate with different countries to help share AACR resources with others.

In Preparation

1. Planning for the unexpected

As an animal-assisted crisis responder, every time I go to a deployment, I am confident of one thing: the challenges that lay ahead, and their respective solutions, will be unique to that particular situation. I know I must be ready for the unpredictable and respond creatively to whatever I encounter at the scene of a crisis. During these times, I remind myself that I am not alone, I am accompanied by Lucy, my best friend and dog partner.

As handlers, preparing our dog team member is crucial. Our overall goal is to control their environment as much as possible to make them feel safe. We also strive to decrease our dog's stress as much as possible, an essential element of animal welfare. One way to ensure the dog feels safe is by preparing the dog for the job ahead and preparing the environment of the crisis to expect the dog. The first step toward preparing the dog is to train it. Dogs need special training to be part of a team that responds to crises, and their training must include therapeutic

*Bjaffe2@mail.yu.edu

techniques and crisis training. In this way, they can be ready to encounter different types of scenes that include loud noises, large numbers of people, unusual smells, and, overall, environments that are foreign compared with what they are used to.

Consistency is an essential element that helps create a safe space for AACR dogs. For instance, every time Lucy and I head to a deployment, I put on her vest so she knows what we will be doing. I even ask her, "Lucy, do you want to work today?" Whenever she sees the vest, she runs to the door, so I know she is ready. Moreover, Lucy knows exactly how we work together; once she has her vest on, she knows she is on duty. For example, I hold her leash only with my left hand (so I can have my right hand free to use at the crisis scene); this provides us with some control over the situation. Lucy also knows to approach strangers only when she has my permission; she becomes attentive to her surroundings and the different people in them and understands the importance of obeying work orders.

It is of utmost importance to find the right balance between preparing to be in as much control as possible, while also being aware that one is entering a scene that is, in the end, unpredictable. Therefore, if we come prepared for the unexpected, we can better control the situation for our dog's and our own safety.

2. Is the scene appropriate and ready for AACR?

It is crucial for me to prepare Lucy to attend crisis and disaster scenes, and it is also necessary to prepare the scene itself so that it is ready to receive AACR. Some examples of preparing the scene for AACR include assessing the scene with the emergency responders who have arrived already and asking them if this scene is appropriate for a dog. This means asking: (i) if the survivors present would feel comfortable being near a dog; (ii) if the place where the scene is taking place is appropriate and safe for a dog; and (iii) checking that there are no other animals present that could cause a problematic encounter with my dog.

Additionally, I ask the emergency responders at the scene to find a safe place for Lucy and to let the survivors know that a dog will be arriving. Once Lucy and I arrive at the scene, we act differently according to the type of situation we are addressing. If it is a relatively small scene with few survivors, I wander around with Lucy to find the people who need us and to whom we can provide comfort. However, if the scene is larger or more complex, and we have no way of controlling the number of people who are at the scene or even of knowing if everyone present is fine interacting with dogs, I might instead choose a corner where Lucy and I will stay, and whoever wants may approach us. In case of larger-scale scenes like these, including terrorist attacks, I usually have my tent set up so that survivors can visit us privately. This set-up allows people a choice and those who do not like dogs do not need to interact with Lucy.

Another essential element to consider is the approval process of AACR teams within trauma scenes. This approval system works differently in each country. While in Israel it is not necessary to receive an invitation from the site in order to arrive with AACR teams (if the organization that manages the AACR volunteers has permission), in the USA, AACR organizations must be officially invited by the chief person responsible for the site at the time of the event (e.g. police officer in charge) in order to provide their services. These logistical constraints, and the resultant delays in offered services, can sometimes be frustrating. In any case, these rules are ultimately in place to care for both the survivors and the AACR teams, so it is imperative to follow them according to the country where we are providing services.

At the Scene

1. Self-care for the AACR team

Self-care is a crucial element of AACR. In order to do a great job, we must know our partner's and our own limits, and we should decompress before we reach those limits. We should also work on providing self-care after deployments for ourselves and our dog. For example, after deployment, I give Lucy plenty of treats and let her rest. For myself, I like to journal about my experiences; this helps me organize my feelings, give them names, and express them. It also helps me record my own journey.

As a handler, I make sure to be aware of Lucy's well-being and her disposition to work. I must ensure Lucy is feeling strong before we attend emergency calls. For instance, if Lucy goes on multiple calls without breaks in between, she may get over-tired, jeopardizing her well-being and our work's effectiveness. Thus, I must provide her with enough rest time in between calls.

I also prioritize Lucy's care at all times, and always consider how my dog will experience the scene where we are going. I ensure that she has a corner where I can take her if she needs a break; I bring her a water bowl and treats, and I make sure that she is not forced to interact with others when she does not want to. With these precautions for her safety in place, Lucy is excellent at her job. When we arrive at a scene, she targets the trauma survivors; she directly approaches whoever needs our help and offers her unique form of comfort. Her behavior often informs me who needs help the most urgently.

2. Caring for our animal partner is caring for the survivors

A crucial part of animal welfare during deployment is to be aware at all times of the dog's body language and be attentive to their stress signs. This will ensure we fulfill the dog's needs (which can include taking breaks, drinking water, eating, and going on walks).

When we prioritize care for our dog partners, trauma survivors can perceive the dog's trust in us and unconsciously understand they can trust us too. At this point, the therapy engagement begins because survivors realize we are there to help and comfort them. Though they do not know us, and it is tough at times of crisis to open up to a stranger, the fact that the dog trusts us provides an opportunity for the survivors to develop trust in us.

This mutual trust demonstrates the importance of securing animal welfare not only for the sake of the animals but for the people whom we treat, as well. If we can prove that we are worthy of trust and that caring for our dog is a top priority, then survivors will break through their barriers and open up to us more naturally, so we can provide them with psychological first aid and comfort.

One specific example was when Lucy and I were deployed to the Surfside building collapse in June 2021. Lucy and I were able to help numerous people as they underwent trauma, including the families of those trapped in the building, survivors who had managed to escape the collapse but had lost all their belongings and their homes, the police, emergency medical technicians, emergency responders, and more. Though we were very busy, I was always conscious of the importance of caring for Lucy (providing her with breaks, walks, and long naps). Whenever I saw in her eyes that she was done for the day, I would stop working and bring her back to the room to rest. Her work in dealing with this disaster was outstanding. Lucy always found ways to approach the people who needed comfort the most. With her interactions, Lucy developed communication channels with the trauma survivors so they could express their pain to a comforting, non-judgmental, living being.

One last consideration is that when conducting AACR work it is critical to be culturally sensitive. In Israel, AACR teams are typically not deployed to scenes where there are Muslims or ultra-Orthodox Jews present. Both groups are usually uncomfortable around dogs because they typically do not have any interaction with them. Interestingly, whenever I have been deployed to large scenes where people from these communities were also present, I often found them very interested in interacting with Lucy. After all, this type of interaction with a dog was a unique experience for them (it might even have been the first in their lives). While it is essential to respect cultural customs, it is also valuable to remain open to the possibility that survivors might contradict these expectations, in which case, we should follow their lead.

Conclusion

AACR is a unique approach to helping trauma survivors. When performing this kind of work, it is vital to consider the safety and welfare of all parties involved, such as the survivors, the handler, and, most importantly, the animal. Caring for our animal partners allows survivors to trust our work and let us help them. More importantly, considering all elements discussed in this chapter when providing AACR is the primary way to ensure we care for our dog's safety and well-being.

Discussion Questions

1. As we care for our animal partner, we must also care for ourselves. How do you think one can maintain this balance in a trauma scene deployment? What signs can you notice in a dog to understand that it needs a break? What signs do you show when you need a break?
2. How would you try to work within local/regional bureaucracy in order to help trauma survivors through AACR? What benefits do you see in following these rules? Do you see any disadvantages to these rules?

15 Innovative AAI Within a Child Trauma Assessment Center

ANGELA M. MOE*

Western Michigan University, Kalamazoo, Michigan, USA

Abstract

This chapter addresses the work of therapy dogs within a child trauma assessment center. Incorporating animal-assisted interventions (AAI) with trauma survivors is a growing field of practice and research; however, with this growth comes the need for deliberate experimentation and adaptation. This is a specialized context for AAI, necessitating experience, education, and a particular skillset related to trauma, for both handlers and dogs.

Context

The types of trauma I refer to here are primarily family based (where children face greatest risk) and come in many forms: (i) neglect (physical, medical, environmental, supervisional); (ii) abuse (physical, sexual, psychological); and (iii) exposure (prenatal and postnatal, to alcohol/drugs, domestic or community violence, criminality, and other toxic stress). In addition to physical injuries or other tangible signs of maltreatment (poor hygiene, untreated ailments, malnourishment), children suffer a range of cognitive, relational, behavioral, and physiological impacts. For instance, children who have experienced physical abuse or witnessed the abuse of other family members may exhibit hypervigilance— a constant state of watchfulness and distrust of people. Children who have been abused or neglected from an early age tend to dysregulate easily, finding it difficult to focus on a task, startling easily, and experiencing rapid mood swings. Others unconsciously dissociate, or zone out, sometimes reliving events they've experienced or witnessed. Many are justifiably withdrawn, depressed, and exhibit post-traumatic stress disorder.

Developmental trauma assessments can help expand understandings of the impacts of maltreatment and aid treatment provision. The Southwest Michigan Child Trauma Assessment Center (CTAC) has been conducting these types of assessments for over 20 years. They rely upon validated instruments to gauge learning potential, executive functioning, language, fine and gross motor skills, visual processing, memory, attention, and social communication. They also conduct fetal alcohol exposure screens, psychosocial interviews, and structured parent–child observations when appropriate.

In May 2021, I and my pack of therapy dogs were added to the CTAC team as part of a pilot study on the efficacy of incorporating animal-assisted interventions (AAI) into assessments. My canine partners included:

- Sunny, a 6-year old golden retriever, a registered therapy dog of 5 years and certified crisis response dog of 4 years (Fig. 15.1);
- Oreo, a 3-year old Newfoundland-poodle mix, a registered therapy dog of 2 years and certified crisis response dog of 1 year; and
- Poppy, a 2-year old Newfoundland-poodle mix (rescued younger sibling of Oreo) and registered therapy dog of 6 months.

The pilot project was very successful and AAI is now a permanent part of CTAC services. The

*Angie.moe@wmich.edu

© CAB International 2024. *Animal-assisted Interventions: Recognizing and Mitigating Potential Welfare Challenges* (ed. L.R. Kogan)
DOI: 10.1079/9781800622616.0015

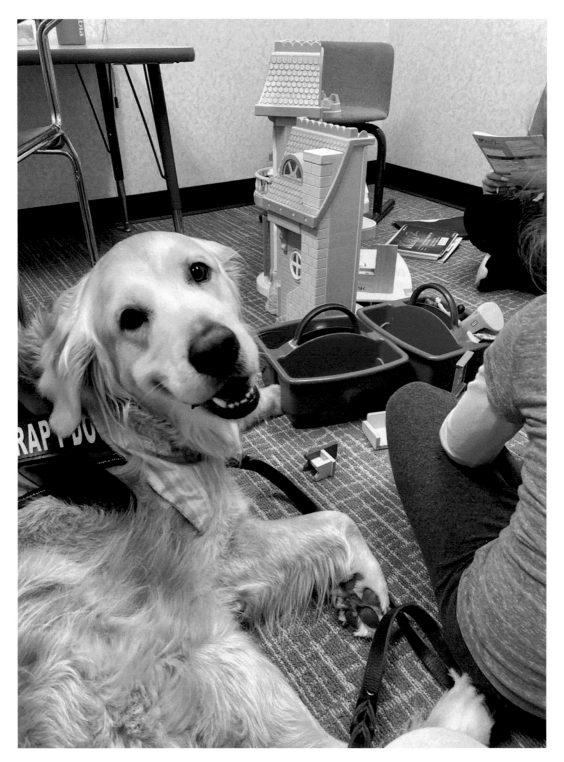

Fig. 15.1. Sunny accompanying a child through testing.

center conducts multiple assessments one day per week, evaluating between five and eight children. I, along with one of my dogs, am present on these days. To date we have assisted in over 350 assessments and logged over 500 hours. The following are my primary observations and recommendations in regard to AAI within trauma-based services for youth.

Experience Matters

The foremost lesson learned throughout this work is the importance of careful animal selection. AAI within this environment, where trauma survivors are receiving services, is largely beyond the skillset or capacity of a typical therapy dog. The nature of the work is more aligned with animal assisted crisis response (AACR), which is a distinct certification reserved for experienced therapy dogs that show an aptitude for working in more fluid settings involving crises and disasters. It involves longer hours, higher emotions, and less predictability. Only experienced and fully mature dogs should be employed in these settings.

To that end, at the start of this project I assumed that Sunny would be the main and perhaps only dog involved with CTAC. He started as a classroom therapy dog in my collegiate courses which often contain sensitive subject matter (similar to that addressed at CTAC), and has many years of experience along with several crisis/disaster deployments. My second dog, Oreo, had been on track for this type of work as well, but the coronavirus (COVID-19) pandemic curtailed his early training. As such, he was introduced to CTAC more slowly and through shorter intervals after the pilot project was well underway. He built up endurance (along with receiving AACR certification) and demonstrated an affinity toward youth (especially among the youngest kids who are prone to dysregulate, as well as withdrawn teenagers). Poppy is just starting at CTAC, for short periods and less frequency. I will not fully engage her until she is at least 3 years old and/or AACR certified.

Experience also matters for handlers. We are caring individuals by definition, and I think we tend to want to help make a difference with every person our dogs meet. It can be easy to miss our dogs' stress signals. Further, therapy dogs, especially the highly skilled ones, have large zones of tolerance. They can handle a lot and their body language tends to be more subtle than other dogs. It is thus critical that we know the types of behaviors our individual dogs exhibit when they are feeling stressed, and honor what we see from them by giving them ample breaks, rest time, and opportunities to decide how they interact and with whom.

Similarly, we must be attuned to our own reactions to situations. Working with trauma survivors often involves learning about extremely difficult things. It is heartbreaking to hear of the ways in which young people are victimized by those on whom they depend. Secondary traumatic stress, sometimes referred to as vicarious trauma, is common. We must recognize that we absorb much of what our dogs experience, even if secondarily. Specific education on trauma-informed practice and mental health first aid are recommended, as is awareness of one's own stress responses and self-care.

Flexible Techniques

Primary tenets of trauma-informed practice include honoring the unique experiences of survivors, and working to find ways to encourage their empowerment and agency. Therapy dogs provide a unique approach to this, since so many will accept attention from humans unconditionally, and are drawn to those who are suffering. I think most therapy-dog handlers who have worked with trauma survivors know that facilitation of their interactions is as important as trusting them to do our dogs work. This is where traditional therapy-dog handling techniques (rules) rub up against intuition.

Many therapy dog organizations encourage or even require the use of shorter leashes (2–4 feet or 0.6–1.2 m), which necessitates remaining in close proximity to the people with whom our dogs interact. Such close personal distance can be threatening for a trauma survivor. It's important to remember that it's our dog they are interested in, not us. Hence, I have found that using a longer lead or dropping the lead, while remaining nearby, provides a great deal more comfort for the children at CTAC and facilitates more organic interactions with the dog. In such circumstances, I try to be discreet in my supervision, moving toward a wall

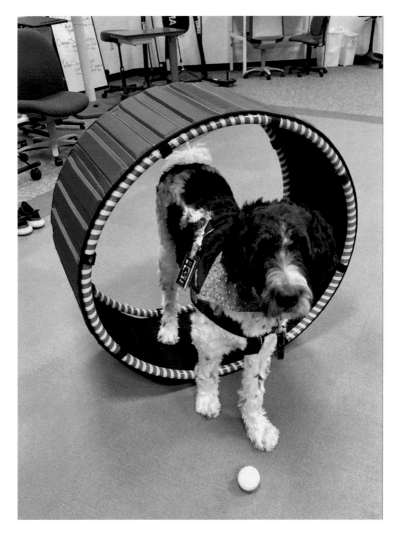

Fig. 15.2. Oreo playing after an assessment.

(so as to be less obvious) and lowering my body to be at or below eye level of the child and dog (to lower spatial hierarchy). I remain present and observant, but not intrusive.

I have found some other carefully monitored off-leash activities useful as well. Two of the most common are inviting kids to walk my dog indoors or play fetch with them down hallways. Many children arrive at CTAC having traveled for some time (up to 3 hours one way) and are understandably anxious. It doesn't help that the environment

is very clinical, resembling a doctor's office or small hospital. As such, the presence of a dog often quells trepidation and establishes a more welcoming tone to the space. Specifically, inviting a child to walk the dog from the lobby to their assessment room provides a nice transition to testing, and offering a game of fetch during breaks helps to ease the tension and fatigue that accumulates throughout the day (Fig. 15.3).

However, for valid reasons, off-leash work is often prohibited by therapy dog organizations.

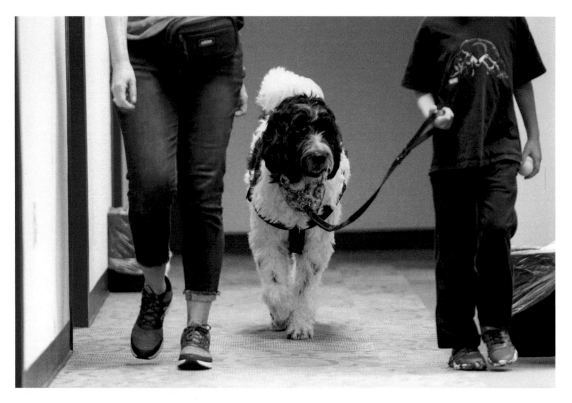

Fig. 15.3. Oreo being walked during a break. Photo courtesy of Western Michigan University Marketing and Strategic Communications.

For comparison sake, however, agencies that employ facility dogs, which may or may not have specific AAI training, seem to have fewer rules regarding leash work. What I have found, within the context of ongoing work with an exclusive group of experienced dogs, is that a middle ground is worth exploring. To be clear, my work with CTAC falls under a grant (it has become part of my job), which replaces the liability coverage I would otherwise receive as a registered volunteer within a therapy dog organization. In other words, I do not represent that organization while at CTAC. I carry supplemental insurance and am also covered by my employer's umbrella policy. Such adaptations are contingent upon understanding what is and is not permissible under particular circumstances, and being very clear about representation. My point is to raise the possibility that within this context, my dogs are blending the roles of therapy and facility animal.

With the many hours we have logged, and strong relationships we have built with the staff, such experimentation and flexibility have aided our efforts to provide trauma-informed care.

Conclusion

This chapter addresses the specific context and challenges involved with incorporating AAI into clinical trauma assessments with children. This is a very specialized context for AAI, necessitating experience, education, and a particular skillset related to trauma, for both handlers and dogs (Fig. 15.5). However, with time, opportunity, and support, much can be learned and developed in regard to evolving the ways we think about and approach AAI with children who have experienced trauma. As the field of AAI advances, such deliberate experimentation may help move our efforts forward in meaningful ways.

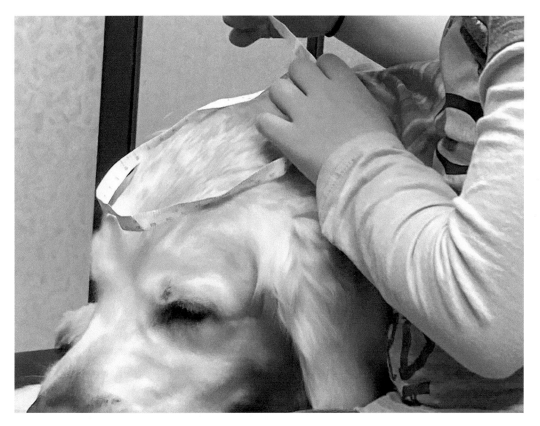

Fig. 15.4. A child measuring Sunny's head in the pediatrician's office.

Case Example I

Emma, 4 years old, is receiving an assessment at the CTAC after being removed from a severely neglectful home. She had rarely been out of the house prior to entering foster care, and misses the various pets she used to have. Emma is excited when told that there is a therapy dog at the assessment center and her face lights up when she meets Sunny. She excitedly walks him down to the room in which her assessment will occur. The clinician working with Emma requests several visits with Sunny throughout the day, even to accompany her to the pediatrician's office. Emma is fearful of the doctor, so Sunny is invited to jump up on the examination table with her. Together the doctor and Emma measure his head (Fig. 15.4) and listen to his heart with a stethoscope. Emma then agrees to have the same done to her.

Case Example II

Jordan, 15 years old, suffered significant physical and emotional abuse by his step-father, as well as witnessing domestic violence against his mother. He was recently arrested for trying to steal a car and is in a juvenile detention facility. He arrives at the CTAC wearing an orange jumpsuit, shackled at the wrists and ankles, and accompanied by two deputy sheriffs. He seems embarrassed and makes little eye contact or conversation, though he does pet Oreo's head upon introduction. During the interview portion of the assessment, Jordan and his clinician sit on the floor in order to be more comfortable (he remains shackled). Oreo sits in on this interview, laying his head on Jordan's lap. Jordan continues to stroke Oreo's head and speaks about how dogs are "man's best friend". He shares his fear for the abuse his mom experiences, which prompts staff to

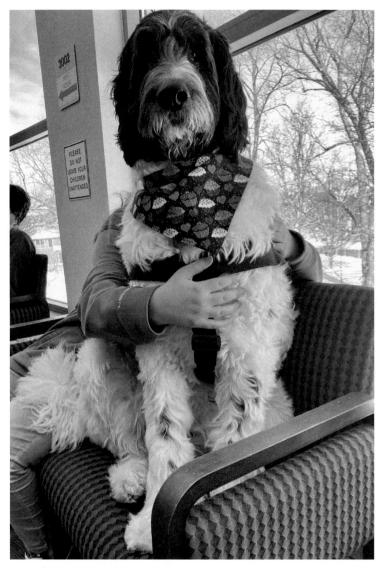

Fig. 15.5. Oreo receiving a hug after an assessment.

recommend specific safety planning recommendations in their report to the court.

Discussion Questions

1. How do you feel about the off-leash therapy techniques described above? Are there other circumstances in which off-leash work could be suitable? What kinds of things should a handler think about before conducting off-leash therapy techniques?

2. The author justifies her approach to AAI as being trauma informed. What does being trauma informed mean to you and how might it apply to contexts in which you may work? How might being trauma informed change the ways you facilitate interactions between your therapy animal and the humans you serve?

A.M. Moe

16 Your Dog to Share

Marin Humane, Novato, California, USA

Abstract

Animal-assisted interventions (AAI) in animal welfare requires training for both the person and their dog emphasizing their relationship. The Your Dog to Share class prepares volunteers and their dogs to serve as animal ambassador teams at Marin Humane. Successful teamwork between the dog and handler requires a strong, bonded relationship based on mutual trust, effective communication, respect, and appreciation. This chapter shares class details and specialized training that successfully prepares guardians to be their dog's advocate while volunteering together.

When I tell people I have been working in animal welfare for over 40 years, in my next breath I joke that I started working before child labor laws, so I'm really not that old. Of my 40 years working in animal welfare, I have spent 35 years involved in animal-assisted programs. Animal welfare isn't just a career for me, it is in my blood, it is my passion, and I feel blessed to have a career fostering the human–companion animal bond through animal-assisted programs.

The highlight of my career has been designing and leading animal-assisted programs. I see animal-assisted interventions (AAI) as a prescription for the human–animal companion bond. That bond is so powerful that simply being in the presence of a companion animal can elicit positive interactions and chemical changes in our brains (Beetz *et al.*, 2012). This unique and magnificent bond is amazing, as I'm sure those of you reading this book have experienced.

Animal welfare in AAI is different from other fields but should, like other practices, adhere to high standards for the animals and their guardians. People are excited about AAI and love the idea of sharing the human–animal bond with others. However, many overlook the animals' needs and the importance of pet guardian knowledge. I have unfortunately witnessed AAI programs at animal welfare organizations that do not prioritize the animal's well-being nor provide training or guidance to their guardians. The program I designed at Marin Humane, Your Dog

to Share, is the culmination of first-hand experience, knowledge, and many years of learning. It is the required training for volunteers and their dogs to become animal ambassador teams and volunteer at Marin Humane (available at: https://marinhumane. org/above-beyond/community-engagement/animal-assisted-programs/ (accessed March 15 2023)). The animal-assisted programming at Marin Humane is diverse, very popular, and well respected in the community. It has had tremendous success because of the training, preparation, and continuing education we provide to our volunteers and their dogs.

If you are interested in sending animal ambassador teams into your community, it is your responsibility to make sure volunteers are well prepared to represent your organization and mission. Volunteers and their dogs can be amazing ambassadors for your organization, but only if they are a confident, skilled team. This takes time and commitment from everyone involved. The Your Dog to Share (available at: https://www.youtube.com/watch?v=T2-rIbA4pww (accessed March 15 2023)) class has developed into a well-oiled training program, bringing a diverse group of people together to prepare animal ambassador teams. The lessons strengthen the human–companion animal bond between the volunteer and their dogs, resulting in a deeper trust and confidence so both can enjoy the work, even when they encounter surprises.

The class consists of six 1-hour interactive lessons, structured to introduce the teams (Fig. 16.1) to new

*Dblackman@marinhumane.org

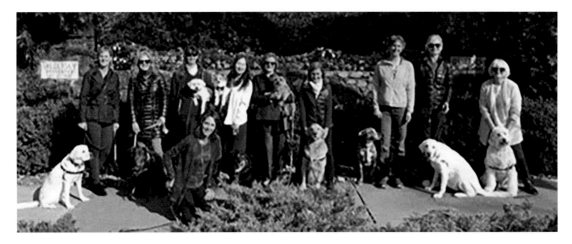

Fig. 16.1. Your Dog to Share graduation.

environments and situations they will encounter in the AAI. These lessons include: (i) learning to read a dog's body language; (ii) safety skills for volunteer and dog; (iii) introduction to medical equipment; (iv) interaction with a group of children; (v) guest speakers; and (vi) field trips that include observation of current volunteers. The last week of class is offsite at a senior community where the new teams experience their first visit, and a graduation celebration.

Prior to the class, interested people receive a list of required skills for their dog. Then a pre-screen appointment is held so the guardian can demonstrate the necessary skills. The prospective team walks around our shelter's campus, inside and outside, while we observe their interactions with people, and people with dogs. We have found that an independent observer is necessary to determine the level of skills and their dog's desire to do the work. Dog training classes teach dogs good manners and helpful skills while strengthening the bond between person and dog. A solid foundation of skills, a strong bond, and a dog's predisposed desire to meet people is a fabulous combination to start with. Additionally, dogs need to be forgiving of odd interactions, recover quickly from being startled, and able to focus on their guardian—even with distractions. If the dog is not agreeable and does not enjoy the interactions, then no one will benefit.

Each week is unique and homework assignments compliment the training. Week one is an orientation to discuss AAI, Marin Humane's programs,

and to learn about each individual's inspiration. The first class together as a group is week two and we observe skill levels and role model visits for each team, demonstrating different techniques related to the dog's size and venue. Week three is the dog body language lesson and this emphasizes the animal's consent. Making sure volunteers understand how to read their dog's cues to ensure their dog wants to interact is key.

The fourth week of class is the most interactive, with different stations set up in different rooms. The dogs will: (i) greet a person in a bed; (ii) visit a person in a chair in a kitchen with food present; (iii) visit with a person who uses a wheelchair (large, electric); (iv) use various cues to maneuver around chairs and past distractions (food or stuffed cat); (v) walk inside and outside using the wait cue at all doors; (vi) watch their guardian use a walker, a cane, and a crutch; and (vii) walk an obstacle course. Feedback is given individually after the obstacle course which is designed to observe the relationship (Clothier, 2002) between the handler and dog. The following weeks include working with a group of children, tricks, veteran volunteers as guest speakers and the Your Dog to Share final, a screening for skills including all the distractions from week four.

Volunteers are reminded to think about their role as the human half of the team. Their dog is *always* the number one priority. There may be times the human needs to change their commitments because of their dog's specific needs that day. We tell them that it is always okay to put their dog's needs first.

D. Blackman

Volunteers are their dog's assistant (booking their assignments), chauffeur, and bodyguard (making sure they are not stressed and guiding people as to the best ways to interact with them). They are half the team, and many times work harder than their dog. If volunteers are close and comfortable, their dogs will feel safe and confident; in turn, giving the team the ability to interact more freely. One of my most common reminders during class is to tell volunteers to remember to praise their dog; appreciation of their efforts also builds trust. The connections teams create can be very intimate and emotional, so being comfortable allows both volunteer and their dog to be open.

One of my pieces of sage advice is to think about the best way to work with your dog; training vs management. Training is "hoping for the best" (no matter how well trained) while management is "setting up for success". For example, to avoid a spill on the floor, you could use the "leave it" or "touch" cue or you could put your body between your dog and the hazard and walk quickly around it while keeping your dog's attention on you.

Case Example I

A new team was assigned to an assisted-living facility. He and his dog were amazing in class and made a wonderful team. He really enjoyed the work and visited once a week. The *no* treat policy was explained and emphasized during class. This policy is particularly relevant when a team is to interact with older adults, who from aging have thinner skin, meaning that even the gentlest dog can inadvertently cause injury when accepting a treat.

The volunteer had watched a documentary about a program that incorporated Cheerios breakfast cereal in the AAI sessions at a senior community. His excitement and enthusiasm regretfully overshadowed his recollection of the no treat policy.

During a visit, one of the residents had a cut on his hand and when he gave the treat to the dog, the dog's mouth rubbed against the cut and it started to bleed. The staff at the facility knew he had a cut and realized that the bleeding was not due to a bite. Yet, later when his family visited, they were upset that he had an injury that had occurred during an interaction with a dog. Unfortunately, their protests led to reporting this incident to public health officials. This involved home quarantine for the dog and great embarrassment to the volunteer. The staff at the facility also felt bad that they had to report

it, they understood it was not a bite. Thankfully the incident did not impact the relationship with this senior community. Sadly, however, the volunteer did not want to continue volunteering, resulting in the program losing a wonderful team.

Case Example II

One of our reading teams was in a public library. The librarian had a very organized program with children signing up for different time slots with our teams. Volunteer teams sat in between shelves to have a private place to read one on one with the children.

During one reading session a child came running into the library and ran around the reader and the volunteer and jumped on the dog. It was upsetting to all, including the dog who, because he was in pain, reached back and nipped at the child's face. The librarian and mother came over and removed the child. They both apologized profusely, explaining that he has a disability, has very little impulse control, and does not understand that he can hurt a dog.

The volunteer removed her dog from the library, examined him to be sure he was not injured and then took him for a walk. He was not injured, and she wisely let him relax during the walk and then brought him back in the library to just walk around and receive praise before leaving on a happy note.

The parents did not want to report the bite and said their child has had this happen before with other dogs. They took full responsibility for their child's actions.

Discussion Questions

1. How might you have handled these situations?
2. What preventative measures might you implement to help reduce the chances of these occurrences?

References

Beetz, A., Uvnäs-Moberg, K., Julius, H. and Kotrschal, K. (2012) Psychosocial and psychophysiological effects of human-animal interactions: the possible role of oxytocin. *Frontiers in Psychology* 3, 234. DOI: 10.3389/fpsyg.2012.00234.

Clothier, S. (2002) *Bones Would Rain from the Sky: Deepening Our Relationships with Dogs.* Grand Central Publishing, New York.

17 Benefits and Considerations when Incorporating Farm Animals in Therapeutic Settings

SUZANNE M. KAPRAL*

The Lands at Hillside Farms, Shavertown, Pennsylvania, USA

Abstract

Farm animals are increasingly incorporated in educational and therapeutic settings. Farm-based animal-assisted interventions (AAI) are methods designed to help individuals, often children, living with trauma, depression, anxiety, and addiction. This chapter explores the benefits and possible welfare implications of farm-based activities for both children and animals. Research supports that humans of various ages and capabilities may benefit from repetitive, structured farm-animal interventions. What is not clear are the effects that repetitive, structured interventions have on farm animals. As the practice of farm-based therapy services grows, we must consider the moral aspects of these sentient beings.

Identifying the Welfare Gap for Farm Animals in Therapeutic Settings

The American Veterinary Medical Association defines animal welfare in part as, "how an animal is coping with the conditions in which it lives". (AVMA, nd). An animal is in a good state of welfare if (as indicated by scientific evidence) it is healthy, comfortable, well nourished, safe, able to express innate behavior, and if it is not suffering from unpleasant states such as pain, fear, and distress. Peer-reviewed studies support the positive outcomes that animal interactions can have on humans (e.g. Enders-Slegers and Hediger, 2019; Rault *et al.*, 2020; Rodriguez *et al.*, 2021). Yet, it is in the best interest of both humans and animals to recognize potential ethical challenge, particularly for farm animals. Depending on cultural perceptions and experiences, individuals may not believe that cows, chickens, goats, and sheep deserve the same level of care or respect as the animals traditionally incorporated into animal-assisted interventions (AAI), such as dogs and horses. An educational dairy farm

located in Northeastern Pennsylvania is working to broaden the scope of farm-based AAI by including how animal welfare corresponds to a healthier, more sustainable society.

The Farm Teaches

The Lands at Hillside Farms (Hillside) is a 428-acre, 19th-century, non-profit educational dairy farm located in Shavertown, Pennsylvania. As the only hands-on teaching farm in Northeastern Pennsylvania, Hillside offers an engaging educational environment not experienced in traditional classrooms. Students work side by side with educators and "co-faculty" farm animals to learn about a sustainable lifestyle, including courses in science, agriculture, ecology, animal husbandry, animal welfare, nutrition, land conservation, and community service. The programs described in this chapter include dairy calves and layer hens with a One Welfare focus that animal welfare, biodiversity, and the environment are connected to human well-being (Garcia Pinillos, 2017).

*Suzanne@thelandsathillsidefarms.org

DOI: 10.1079/9781800622616.0017

The Farm Heals

In 2013, Hillside launched a 3-week long Green Care program to help children better understand feelings and behaviors related to trauma. Hillside Green Care serves children aged 6 through 14 who had a family member die through natural causes, illness, accident, suicide, or homicide. It also welcomes children in foster care, or who have one or more parents in active addiction or recovery. There is no charge for a child to attend. Referrals are received from mental health professionals, social workers, family court, child protection services, guidance counselors, or family physicians. To ensure safety of children, staff, and animals, individuals with a history of violence or self-harm are not accepted.

Green Care includes farm-based chores combined with mental health services. Mental health professionals, trauma specialists, occupational therapists, and registered dietitians facilitate daily individual and group sessions. All farm-staff members facilitating activities receive training in trauma-based care, including compassion fatigue. Staff are required to participate in a farm animal behavior and welfare workshop that includes how human behaviors can affect an animal's physical and mental state.

Farm-Based Programs for Children Who Experienced Trauma

Animals in Hillside's Green Care programs include the dairy herd, calves, goats, pigs, donkeys, and hens. This chapter focuses on calves and hens. Animals selected for farm-based services must be in good health as determined by a veterinarian and show no signs of fear, dominance, or aggression. Hillside does not support the mindset of animals "volunteering" for a session since that indicates choice. Instead, animals must demonstrate "willingness" evidenced by openness to approach without apprehension, fear, or aggression.

Animals are checked each morning prior to children arriving at the barn. An animal exhibiting one or more indicators of fear, stress, or aggression are excluded from the day's interactions. Even in the absence of stress indicators, the burden of responsibility for human safety and animal welfare lies with the humans assigned to their care.

Why is farm-based education a component of trauma services? By working alongside staff, children learn about sustainable agriculture and farm animal anatomy, as well as how animals are used for food and clothing. Experiential learning provides children with a heightened awareness of the importance of respecting the Earth, environment, animals, and each other. Hillside teaches, "why we do" alongside "how we do". In this farm's experience, physical activities performed in fresh air and sunshine appear to reduce stress and increase openness to communicate.

Each day begins with a review of safety practices and rules emphasizing the welfare of children and farm animals. Morning sessions (9:00 a.m. to 12:00 p.m.) are for animal care and afternoon sessions (12:30 p.m. to 3:00 p.m.) include therapy and grief-related activities. Farm-based services are capped at 15 children, with a 1:3 staff-to-children ratio. A staff member must accompany and supervise children while at the farm.

Animal care safety practices and rules:

- Barn tools (shovels, brooms, wheelbarrows, etc.) are to be used as intended and immediately returned to storage after completing chores.
- Children must wear gloves when working inside the barns or with animals. When finished, they should dispose of gloves in designated containers and thoroughly wash hands.
- Sturdy shoes are required. Long pants are recommended. Necklaces must be tucked into the shirt. Bracelets are not allowed.
- Children may not run in the barn or around animals, yell or scream while in the barn. Children must understand that regardless of size, animals have startle reflexes that may include kicking, biting, scratching, and head butting.
- Children may not hover over any animal or approach from behind.
- Children may not hand-feed animals (including human food). Animals may become food aggressive.
- Children are not to chase any animal. Given the species, the animal may feel threatened (hen) or interpret as play (calf).
- After chores, children must return to a designated seating area and wait for others to finish chores.

Calf Nursery

Calves are housed in pairs or groups, except for newborns. Calves arriving in the calf nursery are alone in a pen until determined healthy. The nursery configuration allows for all animals to see and communicate with each other. Being enthusiastic eaters, bucket-fed calves are generally separate from bottle-fed calves.

Staff explain the behaviors of fragile newborn and weeks-old calves to the children. On average, calves are born weighing between 45 lb and 65 lb (20–29 kg), with some newborns weighing 90 lb (41 kg), exceeding a child's weight. An excited calf often runs around the pen, kicking up its back legs. Head butting is to be expected and prepared for. A calf will stomp its foot, swish its tail, and shake its head attempting to rid itself of flies. A hungry calf anticipating feeding can be assertive with bottle sucking or bucket feeding, increasing the risk of a child being pushed or pulled to the ground.

Children work side by side with a staff member at the nursery. No child is ever put in a position of feeding, mucking out stalls, or turning animals out into a field without strict staff guidance and supervision. No child is required to interact with any animal. Safety measures, however, do not reduce the effectiveness of the human–farm-animal connection.

The benefits of such interactions were reflected in the experience of one girl, whose mother died weeks before. She insisted she didn't want to talk about her loss. But while bottle-feeding a calf, she began to talk about passing farms with cows on the way to the hospital to visit her mother. The act of feeding the calf created a safe opportunity for the hurting child to begin sharing experiences and feelings.

Pastured Hens

As a species low in the food chain, chickens have physical characteristics to help protect themselves from predators. Most notably, chickens' eyes operate independently of one another. Simultaneously a chicken can seek bugs on the ground and look for hawks in the sky. Their 300° field of vision—nearly twice that of humans—impacts the way hens experience their environment. Humans walk to a location; chickens *walk into a location*. For example, a person would walk toward a campfire intending to relax and enjoy roasted marshmallows. The hen would be terrified approaching a campfire; she sees the flames as surrounding and consuming.

Hens explore their world by head bobbing and pecking. They peck the ground looking for

bugs and will peck at a person's feet, hands, and legs—a concern if beaks are not trimmed. A child pecked by a curious hen may react by hitting or kicking the bird. Hen behavior is one reason for our clothing rules. Sturdy shoes, long pants and long-sleeved shirts are recommended due to "exploring" hens. Necklaces must be tucked into clothing and bracelets are not allowed as reflecting metals and dangling necklaces or bracelets encourage pecking.

Hen-related chores provide satisfying opportunities for younger or easily distracted children to work as partners or in teams. Filling buckets with grain, changing out water stations, and scattering fresh vegetables and fruits are activities that provide instant feedback. Hens typically run to fresh-food sources and explore vegetables and fruits with enthusiasm. Children who are more focused may work together gathering, washing, and packing eggs for sale in the farm's dairy store. Responsibilities yield benefits including feelings of accomplishment, heightened self-esteem, and trust in another person.

Conclusion

Age-appropriate AAI offers therapeutic benefits when used in the right settings. Farm-based therapy helps provide a calming effect for children while building trust and increasing empathy. Green Care helps teach about the interconnectivity among humans, farm animals, and the environment, all key factors for a healthier and more sustainable future as well as helping children learn to be responsible stewards of the Earth and animals as they heal from trauma.

Case Example I

Discussion questions

1. After studying the photo of the child bottle-feeding a calf (Fig. 17.1), what recommendations would you make to improve the child's safety? Are there any welfare concerns for the calf that can be easily corrected?
2. As you look at the photo of the child with three calves (Fig. 17.2), please identify at least two welfare concerns for the calves and two safety concerns for the child. What are your thoughts on the sizes and weights of the calves?

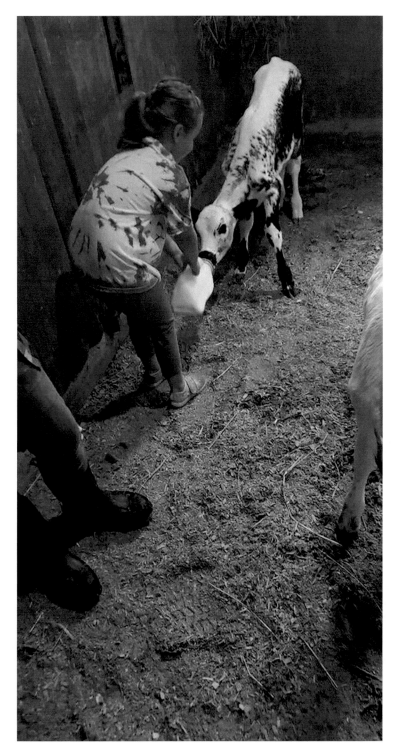

Fig. 17.1. A child bottle-feeding a calf. Photo courtesy of Hillside Farms.

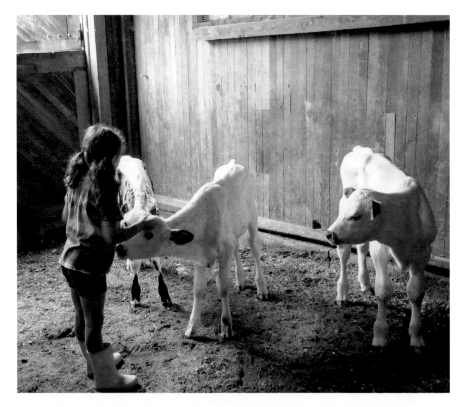

Fig. 17.2. A child at Hillside with calves. Photo courtesy of Hillside Farms.

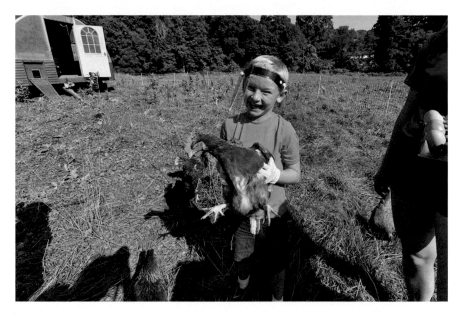

Fig. 17.3. A child at Hillside holding a hen during morning farm chores. Photo courtesy of Aimee Dilger.

S.M. Kapral

Case Example II

A child at Hillside is holding a hen during morning farm chores (Fig. 17.3). The child is wearing gloves as required.

Discussion questions

1. What are the welfare concerns for the hen? How would you improve the welfare of the hen?
2. Based upon your observations, what concerns do you have for the child? What are your recommendations to improve the child's safety?

References

American Veterinary Medical Association (AVMA) (nd) Animal welfare: what is it? Available at: https://www. avma.org/resources/animal-health-welfare/animal-welfare-what-it (accessed 20 March 2023).

Enders-Slegers, M.J. and Hediger, K. (2019) Pet ownership and human–animal interaction in an aging population: rewards and challenges. *Anthrozoös* 32(2), 255–265. DOI: 10.1080/08927936.2019.1569907.

Garcia Pinillos, R. (2017) "One Welfare": a framework to support the implementation of OIE animal welfare standards. *OMSA Bulletin* 2017(1), 3–8. DOI: 10.20506/bull.2017.1.2588.

Rault, J.L., Waiblinger, S., Boivin, X. and Hemsworth, P. (2020) The power of a positive human-animal relationship for animal welfare. *Frontiers in Veterinary Science* 7, 590867. DOI: 10.3389/fvets.2020.590867.

Rodriguez, K.E., McDonald, S.E. and Brown, S.M. (2021) Relationships among early adversity, positive human and animal interactions, and mental health in young adults. *Behavioral Sciences* 11(12), 178. DOI: 10.3390/bs11120178.

18 Animal-assisted Interventions: Paths to Propagation

Julie Ann Nettifee*

NC State College of Veterinary Medicine, Raleigh, North Carolina, USA

Abstract

Any animal-assisted intervention that is successful must include a full evaluation, both initially and continued monitoring, during the intervention to ensure that it is a beneficial intervention for all involved. If the inclusion of an animal at any time causes undue stress, injury, or illness, the detrimental effects to the animal, participant, and program can be substantial. In this chapter, examples of "paths to propagation" are highlighted to ensure the relationship is positive for all involved.

Animal-assisted interventions (AAIs), including many species, can often benefit both the human and the animals. As with any intervention, however, there will only be therapeutic benefits if there is not an increased risk placed on the person receiving the therapy or the animals involved in the process.

As a licensed veterinary technician and specialist in neurology, and as one who has trained others in a variety of settings, I am sharing some "paths to propagation" that I have learned over the years. The word propagation, although in many sectors used only when working with plant species, can apply to AAIs in a powerful way. Propagation is considered both art and science, requiring knowledge, skill, manual dexterity, and experience for success. "To understand the science of why, when, and how to propagate requires basic knowledge of growth and development, anatomy and morphology, and physiology." (Moore, 2018). All these same details can be applied as we support both the animals and the humans involved in AAI.

From my experience and training in AAI, I would like to present a few ideas that have been of great importance and significance to me.

Animal Selection and Monitoring Through the Therapeutic Intervention

There are some studies evaluating the use of purpose-bred versus rescue animals for therapeutic interventions (Thodberg *et al.*, 2014; Fine *et al.*, 2019; Nettifee, 2022). In all cases, however, evaluation of the animal to ensure that it has characteristics to be an appropriate fit for the intervention is critical. In veterinary medicine, one of the mottos is to "above all do no harm". Initial evaluation to monitor and evaluate overall health, behavior, nutrition, and other components are critical to the success of an animal being incorporated fully into an AAI program. Just because an animal is available does not mean that it is a good fit for an AAI program.

---
*janettif2@gmail.com

DOI: 10.1079/9781800622616.0018

Can it be successfully "propagated" into a therapy program? Possibly, with enough nurturing, care, nutrition, and training. Without the above it is a liability.

Case Example I

One case example is Misty, a pony donated to an equine-assisted therapy program that I supported. Misty was older and in need of veterinary care. She was a prime riding pony in her day and had taught many children during her years at a popular local stable. She was donated to a therapeutic equine-assisted therapy program as she could not be used to the extent they needed. As a result of her age, she had developed some difficulty with her vision and arthritis. She needed proper introduction to therapeutic equipment as well as side walkers (people who walk alongside the rider in lessons, who may help the rider with physical support, and encourage or help them to complete a task as directed by the instructor); however, she was gentle and accepting. The program had established a 3-month trial program for all donated animals to assess how well they would fit into the program and determine if alternative options were needed.

Misty worked out well but needed daily care, therapy, enhanced senior nutrition, and continued monitoring throughout the AAI training, which will be highlighted in Case Example II. Although Misty was a purpose-bred pony for show and training needs in her younger years, her highest calling perhaps was as an AAI pony helping children with both physical and emotional challenges reach new heights through the help of this program.

Discussion questions

1. When considering the acquisition of an animal into a program, what method works well to ensure a humane trial/transfer if the animal is deemed to not be a "good fit" for the needs of the program?
2. In the case of Misty with her history, how would you monitor her through the AAI to ensure she remains fit for this type of work?

Case Example II

This scenario involves a canine that was incorporated into a veteran service organization. Dogs utilized in this program are rescue dogs and chosen by the service member. The dogs undergo a behavior evaluation by the executive director or behaviorist to ensure that the dog has characteristics that may make it a suitable fit. This evaluation includes screening for behavior responses to various stimuli and aggression or fear-based responses. Some of the dogs will propagate well, and with weekly training as a group, and individual training by the service member, reach potential for certification for therapy and/or service, depending on the individual's needs.

Buddy was a mixed breed, 2-year-old Labrador that was quite social, eager to take part in training, and overall was believed to be a good fit with the program. One of the goals, however, for this service member was that this dog would provide some physical stability help as their specific disability impacted their neurological balance. Buddy appeared young, strong, and fit. However, after careful monitoring, it was determined that more evaluation was needed for this dog to pass the medical requirements for this specific client. Stability support requires strong hips and back strength and conformation, along with willingness. Buddy had the willingness, yet he did not have the structural ability to help with balance issues. He was, however, able to transition to another handler within the program without these needs, and thereby still propagate his ability to serve to his greatest purpose, while at the same time not incurring harm.

A positive intervention is one that means both the human and the animal are not harmed in the process. "Above all do no harm", but propagate and nurture that which you can through careful selection, proper care, and monitoring. In this way, you can ensure a successful match and a solid lifelong foundation of mutual benefit.

Discussion questions

1. Buddy had health issues that in some cases would have rendered him unfit for the purpose completely. In this case, since he seemed to otherwise be a great fit, how can monitoring throughout the process help him long term?

2. In what ways should a program ensure appropriateness of fit when incorporating animals with possible unknown past histories or training?

References

Fine, A.H., Beck, A.M. and Ng, Z. (2019) The state of animal-assisted interventions: addressing the contemporary issues that will shape the future. *International Journal of Environmental Research and Public Health* 16(20), 3997. DOI: 10.3390/ijerph16203997.

Moore, K. (2018) Propagation. In: Bradley, L.K. and North Carolina Cooperative Extension Service (eds) *North Carolina Extension Gardener Handbook*. Available at: https://content.ces.ncsu.edu/extension-gardener-handbook/13-propagation (accessed 2 August 2023).

Nettifee, J.A. (2022) Impacts of animal assisted therapy. MALS (Master's in liberal studies) graduate research thesis, North Carolina State University, Raleigh, North Carolina.

Thodberg, K., Berget, B. and Lidfors, L. (2014) Research in the use of animals as a treatment for humans. *Animal Frontiers* 4(3), 43–48. DOI: 10.2527/af.2014-0021.

J.A. Nettifee

19 My Ethical Code: Personal Guidelines for Effective Welfare and Safety Practices in AAI

BRENDA RYNDERS*

Animal Hospital of Sebastopol and Sheepy Hollow Sanctuary, Sebastopol, California, USA

Abstract

When conducting animal-assisted interventions (AAIs), practitioners should act in accordance with ethical principles to ensure the safety and welfare of all participants. This chapter will provide an example of an ethical code of conduct that can be used as a guideline for effective AAI creation and implementation. Furthermore, each part of the ethical code is examined in detail and can be tailored to AAI practitioners based upon their scope of practice.

Introduction

As a counselor, educator, and animal-assisted therapy practitioner, it is my duty to ensure that all activities and interventions are designed to promote and protect the welfare of all individuals involved within the therapeutic process. Since animal-assisted interventions (AAIs) utilize non-human animal participants as a conduit for healing, it is essential for practitioners to shift from a human-based paradigm to an all-encompassing model that addresses the impact of AAI service delivery on the non-human animal. When conducting AAI, I have found that the principles of autonomy, beneficence, and non-maleficence are necessary guidelines in assuring that proper welfare considerations are in place. I have personally utilized these principles in my practice of AAI to create an ethical code of conduct that aids in my development of AAIs, with the goal of establishing safety, maintaining participant welfare, respecting non-human animal freedoms, and ensuring that no individuals are subjected to harm.

My Ethical Code of Conduct

Code #1

AAI practitioners always aim to promote the welfare and safety of clients and non-human animal participants involved in the therapeutic process.

Promoting the welfare and safety of AAI participants involves a multitude of factors, including participant screening and assessment, non-human animal selection, consent from *all* participants, proper monitoring, and an appropriate environment for the delivery of interventions. In my experience, I have worked directly with developmental learning centers, foster support centers, and family service organizations to determine which individuals are best suited for AAI services. Since I conduct AAI within a farm sanctuary setting (Fig. 19.1), I will invite participants to the sanctuary for an introduction to the environment and to gauge their responses to the rescued animals who reside at the sanctuary. During this introduction, I review how to safely interact with

*Brendalu2527@gmail.com

DOI: 10.1079/9781800622616.0019

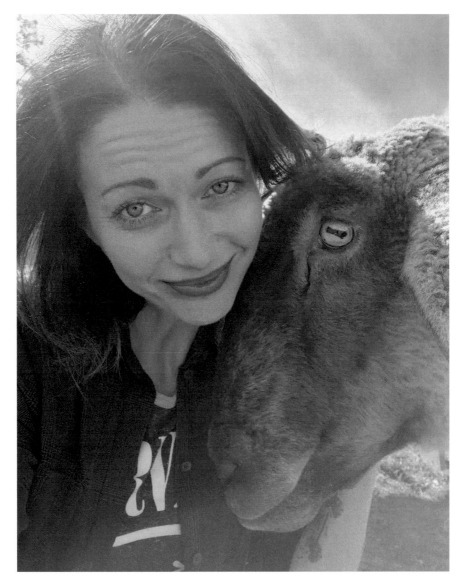

Fig. 19.1. Brenda Rynders with her sheep, Lenny.

the sanctuary residents and carefully observe how the residents respond to each human participant. To me, this introduction is a vital part of the AAI process, as I am able to examine which non-human animal participants are most appropriate in order to have the most effective and rewarding experience possible.

When selecting non-human animal participants, I always focus on individuals who are willing participants and never force any unwanted interactions.

In my experience, I have worked with sheep, cows, goats, and various avian species to forge successful partnerships, foster the human–animal bond, and demonstrate effective boundary setting. Furthermore, I always ensure that all clients are accompanied by an appropriate guardian (such as a parent, social worker, or supervisor from their organization) to aid in actively monitoring participant responses and assist with any mitigation issues that may occur during AAI.

Code #2

AAI practitioners actively aim to avoid actions that would cause harm to clients and/or non-human animal participants.

Safety, in all capacities, should always remain at the forefront of effective AAI implementation. This involves: (i) ensuring appropriate interactions with non-human participants; (ii) active monitoring of participant (both human and non-human) behaviors; (iii) developing suitable interventions based on participant restrictions; (iv) creating a safe physical environment; and (v) providing an immediate response if participant safety is jeopardized. When working with animals, it is essential that participants are engaging appropriately with the animals to avoid harm. For example, practitioners should ensure that human participants treat all non-human animals with respect and compassion by avoiding harmful physical actions (such as slapping, hitting, kicking, or throwing objects) and by using a calm, soft voice when working with their non-human animal partners.

Additionally, it is equally important for AAI practitioners to be actively monitoring the non-human animal participants for any behaviors that could be harmful to human participants, such as head butting or rearing. In instances where harmful behaviors are identified, it is my duty to provide immediate intervention by addressing the behavior and providing an appropriate response. Examples of this would be: (i) physically removing the client from the situation to a new non-human animal group; (ii) working with the client and their guardian to identify risk factors and preventing future harmful behaviors; and (iii) working directly with the sanctuary staff to address non-human animal welfare concerns.

Code #3

The setting of AAI interventions will be appropriate for the client and non-human animal participants.

Another subject of concern pertaining to safety is the environment in which AAI interventions are conducted. Since I implement my AAI interventions in an outdoor pasture setting, I consider how the environment could potentially impact the safety of human participants, especially if there is rough or uneven terrain within the pasture space. Identifying potential risks within the environment is fundamental in maintaining client safety and determining

which interventions can be applied, based on the individual needs of each client. Furthermore, non-human animal participants should always be kept within the safety of their home environment when conducting AAI. One exception to this may be if the non-human animal(s) is comfortable being moved to a different pasture for AAI service delivery if the original environment presented a potential safety risk.

Code #4

AAI practitioners recognize and respect the individual autonomies and umwelt[1] of each non-human animal involved in the therapeutic process.

When assessing non-human animal participants for AAI, practitioners should always allow for the expression of individual freedoms. This includes preparing clients for the chance that their non-human animal participant(s) may not feel social or may not choose to engage in the AAI. Instances like this will happen and have happened to me in my execution of AAI, and practitioners should not become discouraged in these moments. I have found that when this happens, it is in fact a great teaching moment. We, as practitioners, can show clients that non-human animals have their own free will and freedom of choice and if they choose to not engage, that is completely okay.

If I find myself working with a client and a non-human animal who is not engaged, I will shift my intervention to one that does not involve physical contact with the non-human animal, such as meditation and relaxation techniques, playing music for the non-human animal(s), drawing a picture or writing a story for the non-human animal(s), or assisting in cleaning the non-human animal's habitat (barn, pasture, coop, etc.). While these activities do not involve direct non-human animal contact, they can be equally therapeutic and can aid in the development of additional skills, increase self-worth, provide a reduction in stress, and promote a positive mindset in our clients.

Code #5

AAI practitioners recognize and immediately respond to any signs of stress, fatigue, and/or burnout displayed by participants and take necessary action.

Whenever I am engaged in AAI, I am cognizant of any warning signs that suggest a participant (human or non-human) may need a break or may need to conclude the session early. Clients may demonstrate this through physical exhaustion, such as sweating, heavy breathing, or becoming faint or dizzy. Non-human animal participants can exhibit similar symptoms in the form of panting, laying down, or becoming restless. When signs of stress arise, I ensure that immediate measures are taken to ensure that the participant is comfortable, whether that means obtaining drinking water, allowing them to take a break to rest, or by concluding the session early.

Practitioners should also be aware of how weather conditions (hot or cold temperatures) can impact participant presentation. For example, goats are not fond of being wet and will be less inclined to engage in AAI sessions on a rainy day. Similarly, clients may not be comfortable being outside during more extreme weather conditions, so AAI practitioners should be prepared for a change in environment or location if weather conditions present hazards of their own.

Code #6

AAI practitioners practice only within their scope of competence.

By practicing within our scope of competence, we are able to ensure that we are not providing services or interventions that are outside of our knowledge or skill set. Attempting to practice outside of your scope of competence can put both your client and non-human animal participant(s) at risk. In order to maintain the welfare and safety of all participants involved in AAI, practitioners should only implement interventions based on their level of training and expertise and only work with non-human animal participants that they have received proper training with. For example, I have had several clients ask me if they can incorporate horses into my AAIs, but since I do not have sufficient training with horses, I explain that I do not include horses in my AAIs. Involving a horse in an AAI session without receiving proper training could put the horse and my client in an unsafe and stressful situation, which would go completely against my ethical code of conduct.

Case Example

Susie, age 9, presented to an AAI session with her supervisor, Ann, and five other children from a local youth outreach organization. Her AAI practitioner, Jane, has worked with Susie and her group before and is well versed in interventions that incorporate rescued goats into the therapeutic process. Today, Susie and the other children expressed a strong desire to meet some of the goats in a larger herd, whom they have not met before. Since many of the goats in the larger herd are very friendly and social, Jane deemed it appropriate for Susie and her group to meet the larger herd and engage in feeding them treats. Jane had prior knowledge of one larger goat in the group named Billy, who would sometimes become very anxious and would proceed to rear up and ram when feeling stressed. Jane instructed the group to avoid interacting with Billy. As Jane monitored the feeding activity, she noticed that Billy was beginning to exhibit anxious behaviors by pacing back and forth and ramming against a goat that was standing next to Ann. Jane immediately asked Susie, the other children, and Ann to halt their feeding and walk with haste to the entry gate to exit the pasture safely. Once all parties made a safe exit, Jane informed Susie, Ann, and the other children about the behaviors she observed with Billy and the need to leave the pasture. Jane then guided Susie, Ann, and the other children to another pasture to engage in a new AAI activity.

Discussion questions

1. After reviewing the scenario, what do you think Jane could have done differently to maintain the safety and welfare of all participants?
2. Do you think Jane violated any of the codes outlined in the ethical code of conduct? Why or why not?

Note

1 Umwelt is the German word for environment. This word has been adopted by ethologists to mean an organism's unique sensory world.

20 The Three Agendas of Animal-assisted Therapy[1]

EILEEN BONA*

Dreamcatcher Nature Assisted Therapy, Ardrossan, Alberta, Canada

Abstract

This chapter explores the reality of the impact of the human agenda on the animals involved in animal-assisted therapy (AAT). Therapists have a clinical agenda to reach with their client. Clients have an agenda to interact with the animal in certain ways yet animals are sentient beings with their own feelings, wants, needs, and preferences. Ethical AAT practice considers all three agendas and ensures that the animals in practice are both comfortable and receiving enjoyment in all AAT interactions. The chapter explores this concept through two very different case examples.

Ironically, I was going to begin writing the chapter yesterday, but it was a freezing cold –26°C here in Northern Alberta and so my own agenda morphed into having to catch and blanket the horses rather than write about them. It was after I chased them around trying to convince them that the blanket was a good thing that I then came back and had to laugh out loud. Here I was going to write about respecting the animals in animal-assisted therapy (AAT) and the importance of being fully aware of the fact that they have their agenda, which is not your agenda, or your client's agenda. I was going to write about how we need to ethically ensure we are considering all three agendas in the work and not allow our human agendas to lead the session against the animal's will. And then I chased my mini donkey around the property and finally half lassoed him to get his blanket on. I gave up on my Shetland pony and my Connemara because they refused to be caught and so I allowed them to make the choice to not wear a blanket although it was going to be –30°C or below overnight—so who did I do the right thing by? Did I do the right thing by the donkey when I forced him to wear his blanket or by

the two horses I allowed to refuse simply because I gave up trying?

When I think of this in the context of AAT, I think of it on two levels. One level includes the need to 'force' an animal to undergo things s/he may not like or want to do to ensure his/her health and wellness; and the other level pertains to the agenda that we have as therapists for an AAT session. When we bring animals into our AAT practices, we become their advocates, their providers, their ambassadors, and we are responsible for all tenets of their welfare. If we do not catch them to trim their feet, do health and wellness checks, give vaccines or medications, and/or first aid when needed, then we are not meeting our ethical obligation to care for them. But what if they just don't want to work the day your client chooses them in your AAT practice? What if their health and welfare is not at stake and it is more of a mood or a choice to do something else that is influencing their refusal to be part of your session? Are they allowed to say no? What if the AAT session is scary for them or makes them uncomfortable? Does your therapy trump their comfort?

*Eileen@dreamcatcherassociation.com

This is where the three agendas come in. Let's examine the following example.

Case Example I

Josh, a 9-year-old boy, is attending therapy because his mother died and his father is hoping Josh can begin to heal by expressing his feelings through working with your horses. Josh has been to traditional therapy but it has not been effective. Josh is an avid animal lover and his father is hoping that by working with the animals, Josh will feel more comfortable and that an AAT psychologist who specializes in grief work can help him to process his deep grief.

You are that therapist and you have a horse who is very quiet and gentle by nature.

Josh has no experience working with horses and this horse would be perfect for him to begin sessions with. Josh is very excited to brush this horse (Fig. 20.1). When you and Josh go toward

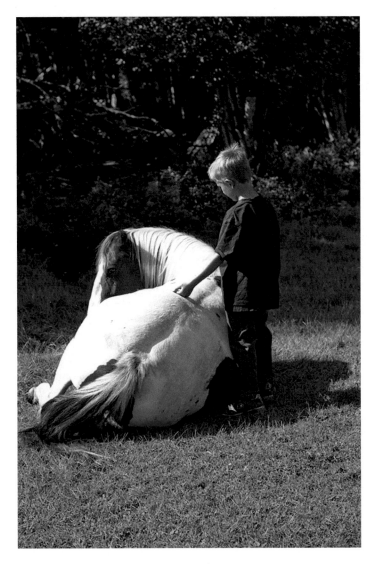

Fig. 20.1. Josh with a horse.

E. Bona

the horse, it turns and walks away, indicating that it may not wish to be caught. Here are three possible agendas at play:

1. Your agenda is to build rapport with Josh through working with your horse.
2. Josh's agenda is to brush the horse.
3. The horse's agenda is to go for a walk, likely toward the food and without you or Josh.

What is the best ethical approach to helping Josh in this moment?

There are many ethical options. First off, you could address the horse's behavior in the context of the horse being a sentient being and having her own thoughts, feelings, wants, and needs. You can ask Josh what he thinks you both should do. This would give you a good indication of: (i) Josh's awareness, understanding, and depth of empathy; (ii) his ability to problem solve; and (iii) the level of his frustration tolerance and many more important social skills. In doing this, you would be meeting your agenda, which is to build rapport and get to know Josh, and you would be meeting the horse's agenda as she gets to go off and eat, but you wouldn't be meeting Josh's agenda as he wanted to brush the horse. Secondly, you could catch the horse and bring her back to brush her, meeting both yours and Josh's agendas but not the horse's.

So how can you meet the three agendas?

Let's say that the horse was going toward the food. Perhaps you can suggest to Josh that he get some food to offer her to see if she will choose to be with him rather than out in the pasture? If she does, then she gets to eat while you teach Josh to brush her and build rapport. All three agendas will have been met!

As a psychologist who has been working in the medium of AAT for 20 years and who offers a certification in AAT and animal-assisted wellness (AAW) to helping professionals, it is my professional opinion that we should always strive to meet the three agendas when working with animals in practice. When we partner with animals, we are partnering with a helper in our work who has their own thoughts, feelings, wants, and needs and we need to notice these, honor them, and meet them as much as is possible. It is unethical to not consider our animal's preferences, likes or dislikes when we are working with them and it is unethical to not adapt our agenda or convince our client to adapt

theirs if these agendas disrespect or dishonor our animals.

Here is another case example.

Case Example II

I was training a group of psychologists from another country on how to integrate animals into their practice. An exercise that I often used to demonstrate the effectiveness of working with animals to help people with frustration tolerance and problem solving was to ask them to catch my llama so that we could explore an obstacle course with her. My llama lives on a 40-acre property and can go wherever she wants to go.

The psychologists' agenda was to catch her. My agenda was to demonstrate how working with animals allows the therapist to conduct a functional assessment of the participants (or clients) while providing the participants with their own insights into their frustration tolerance and problem-solving skills. The llama's agenda was to not be caught under any circumstance (Fig. 20.2).

The psychologists wasted no time planning how they would go about this task and did not ask for help. They all set out with their own agenda to try and catch the llama. They even forgot to ask for a halter or a lead rope! The llama saw them coming, each psychologist fixated on her, directly approaching with the exact predator behavior she avoided. She ran to the farthest side of the pasture with them in hot pursuit. I was definitely getting my agenda met as I mentally assessed each of them for their lack of planning and outward expressions of frustration. I knew the group was going to deeply understand and appreciate the value of AAT for evoking real emotions, providing clear windows of self-understanding, and allowing for teaching opportunities. The llama was getting her agenda met as there was no way they could catch her with that approach. The group was not fulfilling their agenda but more importantly, the llama was clearly not OK with what was happening.

What was the ethical thing to do?

The group were given a task that they were now feeling overly committed to achieve. As I said, they were from another country and their culture had conditioned them to do what they were told and meet the objective regardless of any consequence. It was clear to me that that was the only thing they were focused on. But what about my llama? She was

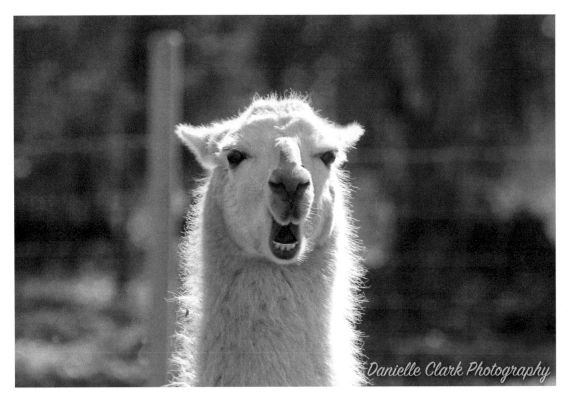

Fig. 20.2. The llama does not want to be caught.

running away from them with her head high in the air and was on high alert for every move they made. Was it fair to her for me to "use" her to teach others in this way? Her agenda to avoid being caught was being met but she was clearly not comfortable with the process. Another part of my agenda was to teach the participants that the animals' comfort and well-being was an integral part of AAT and must always come first. I called time out. The exercise had lasted just under a minute.

I called the group back together and we stood in a circle debriefing what was happening. We discussed how the llama might be feeling, how to read her body language, how they were feeling, what I might be learning about each of them by observing their approach to this, what they were learning about themselves, and most importantly, what to do about the fact that they couldn't meet their objective and that my llama needed to be a mutually consenting part of this process. As we stood in conference, the llama walked up behind our circle and curiously stuck her nose in. Now

that we were no longer acting like predators, she wanted to join our group! The group acknowledged her presence without looking at her and asked if they could get some oats to offer to her. Yes, of course!

They moved together as a group to the oat barrel and the llama followed them and waited patiently over the fence for them to return with the goods. When they returned, they had made a plan to walk to the barn with the oats so the llama would follow to the obstacle course—and she did! They completed the obstacle course, holding a bucket of oats, with the llama walking beside them eating the oats. All three agendas were met: the psychologists achieved their goals, I was able to teach them many important AAT concepts, and the llama was happily content with her new herd. A successful training session for all.

It is important to note that I did not allow the exercise to go on for any length of time so as to not cause undue stress on my animal. It was my ethical AAT duty to stop the process and redirect it to positively include the llama or abandon it altogether if necessary.

Conclusion

I might go so far as to say that we may be oppressing our therapy animals if we coerce them to do what we want because of our personal agenda or that of our client. There are ways to get our animals to share our agenda but often this requires a bit more work. It is our due diligence to ensure that we are checking in on our thoughts, beliefs, and values of animals before we practice AAT and during every single session. If, in fact, we are moving ahead with our human agendas without consideration for our therapy animals' agendas or feelings, then we are most likely practicing animal oppression rather than AAT.

Note

[1] This chapter is adapted from the Dreamcatcher Blog written on January 25, 2021 and titled 'The 3 Agendas of the Triangle Model of Animal Assisted Therapy (AAT)' Available at: https://www.dreamcatcherassociation.com/ourblog (accessed 3 August 2023).

21 Pawsitive Reading Programs

Nicky Barendrecht-Jenken[1]* and Anna van den Berg[2]

[1]Stichting AAI-maatje, Gouda, the Netherlands; [2]Reading Education Assistance Dogs (READ), Salt Lake City, Utah, USA

Abstract

This chapter explores the way the authors work together with dogs in an animal-assisted reading program. An exemplary reading program is one in which the handler and his/her dog share a close bond, a true partnership, instead of using the dog as a tool to get children to read. When handlers have this unique bond with their dog, and the dog truly is given a voice in the interaction, that is when the magic happens.

Pawsitive Reading Programs

Reading Education Assistance Dogs (R.E.A.D.® but hereafter referred to as READ) is an educational reading program for children that includes the opportunity for children to read out loud to a furry friend (Fig. 21.1). The program was developed by Intermountain Therapy Animals (ITA) in 1999 and was designed especially for libraries and schools. In March 2023, there were more than 7000 teams worldwide (in all states of the USA and 27 other countries around the world). A team consists of a handler and his/her own dog (or other furry partners including horses, cats, rabbits, guinea pigs, etc.). The program was developed for children from 6 to 9 years old, but basically everyone who loves to read or has difficulties with reading out loud can join the program.

In the Netherlands, Stichting AAI-maatje (Animal-assisted interventions (AAI) Buddy Foundation) has been working with ITA since 2019. Our teams consist of a well-educated handler and his/her certificated therapy dog. In addition to running the READ-program, Stichting AAI-maatje also offers courses in AAIs and dog-assisted education and reading for those who want to work with their own dog in AAIs.

The challenges

Since the beginning of Stichting AAI-maatje, we have faced several challenges. At first, it was hard to convince people of the benefits of dog-assisted reading. Not only did we have to deal with teachers who didn't believe in this kind of reading assistance, we also had to deal with people's fears including: (i) fear of the unknown; (ii) fear of more work; (iii) fears about hygiene, allergies, cleanliness; and (iv) fear of dogs. Yet, we persevered in spreading the message about the potential of our program. Over time we found several libraries and schools willing to implement a few reading sessions. The results were overwhelmingly positive.

In addition to the challenges we experienced at the beginning, we also had to deal with the coronavirus disease 2019 (COVID-19) pandemic. For close to 2 years, due to the pandemic, we were unable to enter schools and libraries. Fortunately, some of the activities could continue with a face mask and strict hygiene and social distancing regulations, and some activities were able to be conducted online (e.g. reading to our dogs online). Although this was a big difference from the normal face-to-face sessions with the children, it served as a viable substitute. When the government relaxed the COVID-19 restrictions,

*Corresponding author: Info@aai-maatje.nl

DOI: 10.1079/9781800622616.0021

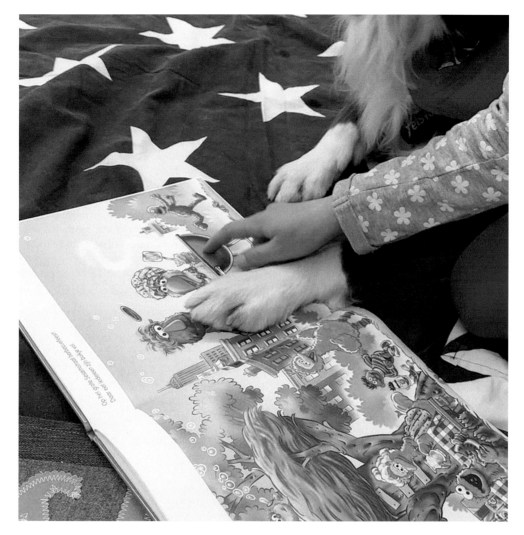

Fig. 21.1. Therapy dog and child in the Reading Education Assistance Dogs (READ) program.

we were able to begin building our program back up. However, one thing never wavered during the pandemic: our enthusiasm and the desire to show and teach everyone about the need for ethical welfare-minded care for the dogs in animal-assisted education.

Interestingly, the pandemic also led to new opportunities. Since the pandemic, schools have struggled with significant learning gaps among students and have started looking for ways to overcome these challenges. We have found that this makes many schools more open to new possibilities.

The dog and handler—like a pair of scissors

Not every dog is a suitable partner for reading sessions with children. It is important to consider the individual dog's traits. The most important character traits are that the dog likes attention and interactions with humans, likes to listen, and is able to keep calm during a session. In other words, the dog should not be too sensitive to stimuli and must have good social skills. Dogs that can be our furry colleagues should feel comfortable in different environments and should not become overly stressed when something unexpectedly happens.

The dogs can certainly be distracted or momentarily startled by sudden noises, but they should be able to recover quickly. Of course they do not deal with any of these situations alone, they always have their handler there to calm them down and help support them when something happens. To be able to be the best handler, friend, and advocate for your dog, we believe that you should be knowledgeable about dog body language and dog welfare. The dog must be able to count on its handler to make sure the situation is under control, and know that their handler will keep their welfare a priority. Only when all parties are safe, can the intervention truly work. The dog and handler can be seen as a pair of scissors: they only work well when both blades are tied together. When one of the blades isn't working, the cut won't be as clean as could be. It is important to be your dog's advocate when working together and give your dog a voice in all interactions.

Circumstances and the dog's well-being

When a new school or library wants to implement a READ program we talk about space, place, and time. What can the school/library expect from us and what do we need from them? What can we do to make the experience as magical as can be for all parties involved? Is there a place the dog and handler can set up their reading space? It is important for the READ program to have a quiet place where children can read undisturbed, but can still be observed. Teams bring their own reading blankets, big enough for all those involved (child, dog, and handler) to sit on (Fig. 21.2). They also bring information explaining the program for visitors and participants. We help our teams prepare their environment, but we also urge them to think about their needs before signing up for a session in a particular place. As their dog's best advocate they

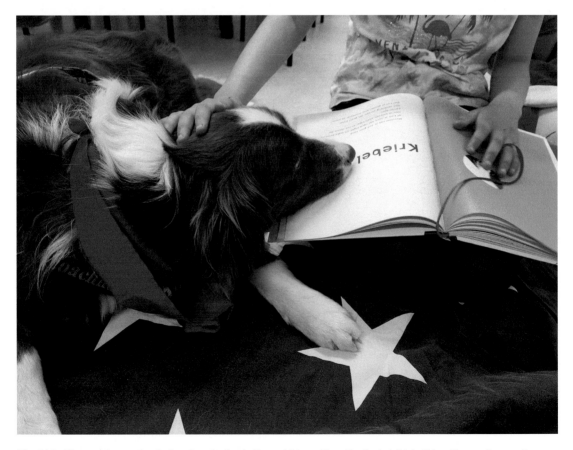

Fig. 21.2. Therapy dog resting its head on the book. Dog, child, and handler (not visible) sit together on the reading blanket.

N. Barendrecht-Jenken and A. van den Berg

know the needs of their own dog best. When the animal feels comfortable, then everyone can feel comfortable. A calm and relaxed dog creates a calm and relaxed environment for a child (Fig. 21.3).

We think it is important to pay attention to the circumstances in which the team will work when setting up a READ program. In addition to paying attention to the circumstances, it is also important that the handler constantly monitors the dog's well-being during the session. This means that when the handler sees the dog is not enjoying the interaction or shows stress signals, they should help the dog feel comfortable or stop the session if needed. Only when the handler knows how to read and respond to their dog's stress signals, can the welfare for both dog and humans be protected.

Case Example I

A certified therapy dog who derives great satisfaction from reading with children is traumatized by a storm. Despite the trauma, the dog still loves to read with children, but is anxious when it is windy outside.

Discussion questions

1. What do you think about this? Is this particular dog able to participate as a reading partner in a READ program?
2. What kind of characteristics should a dog have when involving him in AAI? When do you make the decision to not include a dog or team in AAI?

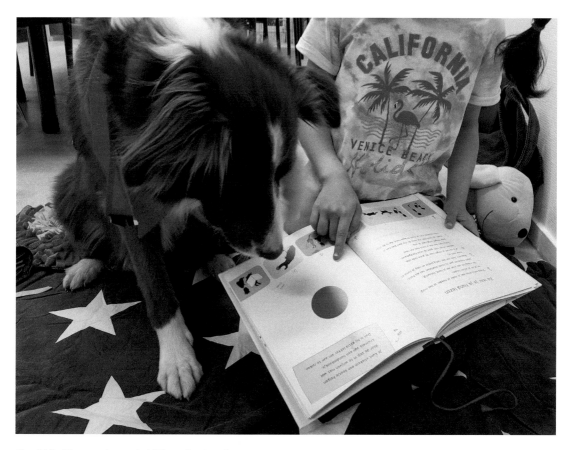

Fig. 21.3. Therapy dog and child reading together.

Case Example II

A school has started a READ program and one of the participating children is a 7-year-old boy. Every week the boy looks forward to reading to the dog. After a few sessions the handler notices that her dog shows more stress signals during the sessions with this boy than during other sessions.

Discussion questions

1. What should the handler do? How can you protect both welfare of the dog and the child?
2. How do you respond to stress signals that your dog shows you?

N. Barendrecht-Jenken and A. van den Berg

22 A Dog's Intuition

Brittany Panus*

West Lane Elementary, Jackson, Missouri, USA

Abstract

This chapter explores a dog's intuition and how certain tasks cannot be taught. Dogs can be taught to sit and stay, but what happens when the things they've been taught are unsafe in certain circumstances? Understanding a dog's intuition can provide insight into how to best support the bond you have with your canine partner. A better bond produces a higher level of trust and a higher level of trust will create a great partnership.

My name is Brittany and I'm a school counselor. My goldendoodle, Layla, works full time with me at two different elementary schools (Fig. 22.1). We also volunteer for local events to create and maintain a presence in our fairly small, rural community. Many community members know us through our work and Layla's sense of fashion. She has a closet full of fun bandanas to match every occasion and her infamous hair bows.

I got Layla with the intention of training her to be a therapy dog. We started training classes at 6 months old and also partook in trick classes as a fun way to bond. We have traveled to several states and enjoyed hiking, swimming, and lunches on fun patios. She is easy going, reliable, and predictable. She knows what my expectations are, and we have a great sense of communication. Our bond is very strong, and I credit our successful work to that. Layla did not start working with me until she was 3 years old. Studies show that dogs do not hit social maturity until they are 2 years old, so we took our time. Her official training was done before she was 1. We then took a couple years to practice and become stronger in a variety of settings and circumstances. I credit that time to our successful partnership, too. We are a registered team through Pet Partners (a national non-profit therapy animal organization) and follow their protocol of only actively working for 2–3 hours per day. So while she is at work all day with me, she is only actively with students for 2–3 hours per day on average. Otherwise, she is secured to a locked drawer in my office with enough space to move around to make herself comfortable to sleep and with access to drinking water. She has done well napping when she is in there alone, which is pretty often some days. She is able to rest and recharge to be at her best.

Service dog teams use a term called "intelligent disobedience" to describe when a dog goes against direct instructions of the handler in order to keep themselves safe. Many, including myself, argue that this ability cannot be taught. Some dogs understand the concept and others do not. My youngest dog does exactly what I ask of him. He does not understand that disobedience in certain circumstances is okay and justified. Layla, however, does grasp this concept. One example happened with a student at school. When walking the halls of my school, Layla walks in a perfect heel to my left. She knows not to leave my side and to keep her attention on me. I taught my students to always ask before petting her because there are times when we can't stop to say hi as I attend to various types of crises in our building. One daily task that Layla accompanies me on is dismissal duty at the end of the school day. We start in the library to dismiss the walkers and then we walk to the bus dismissal doors to say goodbye to students there. One day when Layla and I were headed to the bus doors, we came across a student having a meltdown. This student can become

*Brittanylp92@gmail.com

DOI: 10.1079/9781800622616.0022

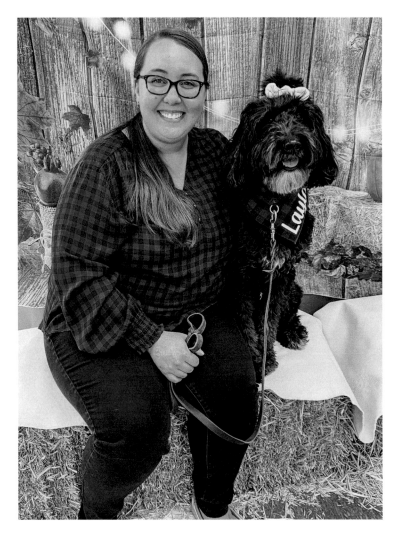

Fig. 22.1. Brittany and Layla sitting together.

violent in meltdowns if she is not well de-escalated. The student was with a paraprofessional who was struggling to de-escalate and looked at me with eyes of desperation. I dismissed the para and took over. This student was kicking and punching and scratching me on top of screaming in my face. Let me preface, this student was not being malicious. She struggles with emotional regulation and we work hard to help her gain skills for coping with disappointment and changes in routine. Her behavior was an outward expression of how she was feeling internally to a last minute change from car rider to After School Kids Club. She was confused, upset, and angry. Now Layla usually walks to my

left side in a heel. As we approached the student, she made the decision on her own to walk behind me to be out of the way. She did not show signs of stress or fear (she deals with screaming students on a semi-regular basis with no issues). I knelt down to be eye to eye with the kindergartner and Layla put herself in a down stay behind me. She had her head on the ground, very settled, and unbothered. I did not teach Layla to do that. I did not teach her how to handle me being hurt. She is very bonded with me and outside of school can be very protective of me and our property. However, in that moment she inherently knew to stay out of the way so I could attend to the distressed student. This kept her safe and it allowed me to do my job uninterrupted. She had an intuition I cannot teach even if I wanted to. Going back to the bond I talked about previously, I encourage therapy dog teams to take their time to get to know each other in various settings. That bond will help support the dog's intuition. In this situation, Layla knew she would not be in trouble for disobeying because we have a strong bond and she can read me like I can read her. I know her signals for stress and fear and I respond accordingly to set her up for success. She trusts me and I trust her, but that took time. I see many teams start working as soon as their training is done. The training may be done, yes, but the bonding and trust may take longer.

There is another set of circumstances where I have witnessed Layla using her intuition. As a school counselor, my office is the host for many upset students. We have seen many tears and many tantrums in our time there. Somehow, Layla knows when it is a good time to offer her comfort services. When I have visitors (adults and students) she stays behind my desk. She does not get up. Sometimes she lifts her head up to see who it is but normally she puts it back down after a brief moment of interest. When I walk away from my desk to meet with students at my table, she remains sleeping behind my desk. There have been several times when I have worked with an upset student. Sometimes they try to mask their feelings, but I can hear it in their shaky voices. I think Layla can too. When we have those moments, Layla will often get up from behind my desk and move to the side of my desk for a better view of the table and just sit there. She won't make a sound. She just sits quietly and observes us at the table. When the student spots Layla, they often ask if they can go say hi or if she can come sit by us. It is very rare that I say no because in my experience, Layla's presence breaks down barriers and helps them feel able to share what is really on their mind. We get to the root of things so much faster when Layla joins us. She creates a bridge of trust that I can't accomplish as quickly on my own sometimes. Her quiet, non-judgmental presence is just the thing they need to show bravery and vulnerability in a way that is often scary and uncomfortable. Yet, she does not get up and sit at the side of my desk every time I work with a student at the table. It seems to only be when she hears the quiver in a student's voice and seeks us out to provide comfort. I am thankful that she has this intuition that sets her apart from so many dogs. Again, I encourage teams to take the time needed to allow that bond and trust to blossom.

Discussion Questions

1. Have you recognized intuition in your dog where you see an unspoken understanding of one another? How can you continue to allow that intuition to grow? What can you do to show your dog they are safe to develop that intuition? Sometimes it means allowing your dog to misread the room or situation safely without harsh consequences.

2. In what ways do you allow your dog to be a dog? Is their off time more than just being at home? Do they get to go on adventures outside of "working" with you?

23 Establishing an Animal-assisted Therapy Program at a Preschool

KATRINA WINSOR*

The New Interdisciplinary School, Yaphank, New York, USA

Abstract

It doesn't get much cuter than kids and dogs, does it? However, it's not as simple as bringing dogs into a school and expecting magic. A successful school-based animal-assisted therapy program requires careful planning and consideration from a wholistic perspective that includes the needs of human participants, service providers, and animal partners. Obtaining the proper training for all staff involved is essential to ensure ethical and effective treatment sessions. This training should include ways to structure programs and sessions that provide the animal participants with freedom to choose to participate (or not) and a schedule with ample breaks and opportunities to relax.

The Pet Pals program in New York, was developed in 2015 to address the need for increased opportunities to incorporate animal-assisted therapy (AAT) into an existing preschool model. Previously, the school had utilized occasional visiting volunteer teams registered through national not-for-profit organizations. Driven by an interest from the staff, it was felt that students could benefit from more frequent and formalized interactions. Therefore, the school sought to develop and establish a structured program to include regular opportunities for animal-assisted interactions (both informal animal-assisted activities (AAAs) and formal AATs).

Initially, several volunteer handler and animal teams agreed to visit the school on a regular schedule. Support for and interest in AAT grew within the school, but the staff and volunteer handlers were unsure how to best proceed with incorporating the dogs into sessions.

At this point, the school decided to seek help from someone who could develop and implement a formal AAT program. One potential welfare challenge to incorporating AATs into a school is ensuring that all individuals have the competency to provide such services, via specialized knowledge and skill development (Trevathan-Minnis *et al.*, 2021). While AAT programs are increasing in popularity, until recently there hasn't been a credentialing program available. The Association of Animal-Assisted Intervention Professionals (AAAIP) was created in 2022 to help address this need (available at: www.aaaiponline.org (accessed March 1 2023)). There is now a certification (the first of its kind) offered to individuals seeking to incorporate animal-assisted intervention (AAI) into their scope of practice (AAAIP, 2022).

AAT Training

For anyone interested in incorporating AAT into their professional practice at a school, they should first ask whether they have the professional knowledge, skills, and experience to offer AAT services ethically and competently. Many therapists are appropriately licensed and credentialed to work within the scope of their disciplines, but do not have any formal training or experience in AATs. The volunteer handler and dog teams originally at the school were all registered through non-profit organizations specializing in visitation for short

*Katrinaw@niskids.org

© CAB International 2024. *Animal-assisted Interventions: Recognizing and Mitigating Potential Welfare Challenges* (ed. L.R. Kogan)
DOI: 10.1079/9781800622616.0023

periods of time, and most often they engage in AAAs during the visits. They had not received formal training in AAT. Additionally, the teams were conducting visits on a voluntary basis leading to occasional scheduling conflicts and cancellation of visitations. Since there was an interest in offering AAT on a regular basis at the school, the administration sought outside help to assist with developing and overseeing an AAT program. The school hired someone who: (i) was in the process of completing a master's degree in applied behavior analysis (with a focus on companion animal behavior); (ii) had completed a certificate course in AAIs; (iii) was a certified professional dog trainer-knowledge assessed (CPDT-KA) and certified behavior consultant canine-knowledge assessed (CBCC-KA); and (iv) had over 7 years working for a professional organization that trained and placed dogs for service work with individuals with disabilities as well as with professionals seeking to incorporate AAI into their practices.

As part of the initial program development, information was collected on the current practices, staff and volunteer experiences, and future goals. All staff were provided with several in-service presentations about dog behavior, training, and AAIs in general, with a focus on AAT. Given the high interest from multiple therapists across several disciplines, it was decided that utilizing a diamond model would best meet the needs of the setting (Jones *et al.*, 2019). In this model, each professional would be able to focus on the student while the animal handler would be able to focus and support the animal. While this model does require good teamwork between professionals to ensure they are on the same page in the activities they will be engaging in, it can avoid the need for the treating therapist to juggle the needs and support of both the student and the animal. Also this allowed each professional to be the subject-matter expert and work within the scope of their knowledge and skills. Over the years, our animal professional has continued to seek out additional education and training opportunities through workshops, conferences, and staying up to date on current best practices through published literature. Ongoing educational opportunities are also provided to all therapists interested in engaging in AAT at the school.

The diamond model used by the Pet Pals program allows AAT opportunities to be offered across multiple disciplines (counseling services, as well as occupational, physical, and speech therapies).

This means that a larger population of students can benefit from participating in an AAT session, but it also means that schedules had to be carefully considered and monitored to not overwhelm the handler–dog teams. Another potential welfare challenge for AAT in a school setting is burnout. While staff burnout is certainly a potential and documented concern within the education profession (Saloviita and Pakarinen, 2021), less is understood about the burnout that the animal partner might experience, particularly if they are working in the school daily. When we go into our chosen vocation, it is exactly that—a choice. In contrast, it might be more accurate to say that animals are conscripted into the profession. This is not to say that this need be an unpleasant experience for the animal; in fact, in a successful AAI program the animals should be willing partners and participants. Instead, the point is brought up to underscore the value of having choice. When there is less choice offered, there is higher potential for negative welfare implications (Nicol *et al.*, 2009). Recognizing that animals are not able to choose to go into this line of work, it is incumbent upon us to safeguard their welfare.

AAT Program Structure

Another important question that needs to be carefully considered, prior to an AAT program implementation, is how will the program and interactions be structured so that the animal partner(s) have ample time to relax and recharge between sessions.

Since its inception, the Pet Pals program has always had multiple canine partners who are able and ready to join in the therapy sessions. In this way, each dog's caseload can be managed to avoid overscheduling which can lead to fatigue or a decreased interest in interacting. The program has a small office that has been designated specifically for the dogs when they accompany their handler to school. The office is set up as a student-free space and is not shared with other staff members at the same time the dogs are present. The room is furnished with dog beds, water bowls, and appropriate toys for solitary dog play. This room serves as a safe zone for the dogs, all therapy sessions occur in other designated rooms.

When a student is considered for AAT the process of inclusion comprises: (i) information from the treating therapist as to why they are seeking to incorporate AAT with this student, including the goals they hope to accomplish; (ii) a background check of the student to ensure there aren't any contraindications for participation in AAT (e.g. allergies, fears, or religious or cultural beliefs); (iii) an initial informal interaction between the student and a program dog to assess interest and compatibility; and (iv) written parental consent for participation. Once a student has gone through this process for inclusion they are matched up with one of the dogs that has the skills and personality that complement the goals established by the student's individual education plan (IEP) goals for the therapy.

At the preschool, therapy sessions are scheduled in 30-min increments, therefore this is the schedule that the Pet Pals program has adapted to. The role of the animal professional is to ensure that each dog has a manageable caseload. When assigning different dogs to participate in sessions, their schedules are coordinated so that they are not asked to participate in back-to-back therapy sessions. Caseload is also assigned based upon the age and experience of each dog: young dogs that are newer to the program and older dogs carry lighter caseloads and are provided more breaks between working sessions.

Additionally, we work to ensure the dogs assent to participate. Assent is obtained prior to the start of each session by the animal professional asking the dog scheduled to work "Do you want a turn?" with their designated working vest being held up in view. This is not an interaction where the dog has been taught to respond with a specific response. Rather, this interaction is designed to provide the dog with some level of control and a means to assess their willingness to participate. This option to participate is offered regularly to each dog and the response differs based upon circumstances and interest. Other examples of this include: (i) "Do you want to go outside?"; and (ii) "Do you want to go for a car ride?" In different scenarios, the dogs have been observed by the animal professional to respond differently, suggesting that they are exercising their right to choose to participate or not in the described activity. Should the dog that was asked for a turn not stand up or approach to be dressed in the vest, this is interpreted as declining to participate in a session. Another canine with the requisite training for the upcoming therapy session would then be asked if they would like a turn for that session.

In the 8 years of the Pet Pals program, there have been many success stories and heartwarming experiences. In part, this is the result of developing and implementing a program that takes a wholistic perspective of welfare. Properly trained staff who continue to engage in professional development allows the program to continuously evolve to meet the changing needs of the preschool's students while adjusting to adopt best practices. Considering the dogs as integral members of the team allows for development of a program and interactions that include positive aspects of animal welfare. Regardless of the species, success in a program is accomplished when an individual: (i) has been properly trained for the job; (ii) understands the expectations and goals; (iii) has the experience and knowledge to be successful; (iv) has the support of all team members; and (v) enjoys engaging in the work that they do.

Case Example

Students are often referred to the program due to difficulties in connecting with the therapist, a lack of compliance to directions, or motivation to participate in traditional sessions. Data collection has shown that students routinely make progress in AAT sessions as compared with traditional sessions. When staff are absent, therapists must make up missed sessions. AAT sessions are carefully scheduled and often fill quickly at the start of the school year. Accommodating reschedules could mean dogs working more sessions than usual on a day or working back-to-back sessions. If AAT sessions are not rescheduled, this means that a student will miss the chance to work with the dog that week.

Discussion questions

1. How do you decide which priority is greater—student or animal?
2. What are the ethical concerns?
3. Do the benefits to the student outweigh the drawbacks of changing the dog's schedules?

References

Association of Animal-Assisted Intervention Professionals (AAAIP) (2022) Certification benefits and fee schedule. Available at: https://www.aaaiponline.org/certificationpage (accessed 3 March 2023).

Jones, M.G., Rice, S.M. and Cotton, S.M. (2019) Incorporating animal-assisted therapy in mental health treatments for adolescents: a systematic review of canine assisted psychotherapy. *PloS ONE* 14(1), e0210761. DOI: 10.1371/journal.pone.0210761.

Nicol, C.J., Caplen, G., Edgar, J. and Browne, W.J. (2009) Associations between welfare indicators and environmental choice in laying hens. *Animal Behaviour* 78(2), 413–424. DOI: 10.1016/j.anbehav.2009.05.016.

Saloviita, T. and Pakarinen, E. (2021) Teacher burnout explained: teacher-, student-, and organisation-level variables. *Teaching and Teacher Education* 97, 103221. DOI: 10.1016/j.tate.2020.103221.

Trevathan-Minnis, M., Johnson, A. and Howie, A.R. (2021) Recommendations for transdisciplinary professional competencies and ethics for animal-assisted therapies and interventions. *Veterinary Sciences* 8(12), 303. DOI: 10.3390/vetsci8120303.

24 Children Interacting with Dogs: Challenges and Rewards

Lisa-Maria Glenk*

Messerli Research Institute (Comparative Medicine) and University College for Agricultural and Environmental Pedagogy, Vienna, Austria

Abstract

The past decades have been characterized by a significant rise of visitation dogs that attend schools and school-like environments to support children's health as well as emotional, social, and cognitive skills. In this chapter, a selection of common difficulties associated with therapy dog visits in schools and school-like environments is presented. Frequent challenges include close physical contact with the dog, gathering informed consent, and pre-instructing recipients. In addition, adequate supervision of the pupils and mindful presence of the responsible person are essential to safeguard animal welfare. Finally, strategies to reduce arousal and to promote calm interactions that support mutual well-being for dogs and recipients are discussed.

Introduction

During the past decades, the popularity of dog-assisted interventions (DAI) designed to support children's physical and emotional health as well as their social and cognitive competencies has significantly increased. Within recent years, canine visitation programs have been incorporated into numerous schools and similar environments. The programs typically seek to improve emotional well-being, cognitive skills such as reading or arithmetic, or to promote safe child–dog relationships by teaching children how to safely communicate and interact with a dog. School environments and specifically children recipients may be challenging for even the best-trained therapy dogs. This chapter provides a selection of common challenges associated with therapy dog visits in schools and school-like environments, based on my 12 years of practice and research experience.

Pre-Instructions and Informed Consent: Preparing Children and Adolescent Recipients with the "Where to Pet Map"

Establishing guidelines to safeguard the dog from overwhelming social intrusion is vital for each dog–child encounter. These guidelines need to address how children can approach the dog, how to behave in their presence, how to appropriately initiate and maintain contact, and how to recognize body areas where the dog prefers to be (and not be) petted. The practical experience I have gathered in more than a decade conducting research and practical programs in DAI reveals that when children want to approach and touch a dog, they often reach out for the head, paws, or tail. However, most canines respond to such advances by displaying appeasement gestures or withdrawal—thus, acting naturally according to their species. To visualize body areas of comfort

*Lisa.molecular@gmail.com

© CAB International 2024. *Animal-assisted Interventions: Recognizing and Mitigating Potential Welfare Challenges* (ed. L.R. Kogan)
DOI: 10.1079/9781800622616.0024

or dislike, a "Where to pet map" can be helpful. Such a map can easily be drawn using a dog's body silhouette that is painted in color according to the traffic light scheme, where red indicates *stop* (these body parts should never be touched), yellow *careful* (representing areas where the dog may not always enjoy being petted and thus, increased attention on stress-related behaviors is warranted) and green *OK to go* (high comfort zone where the dog is likely to enjoy tactile contact from most people). For many dogs, red areas would include the paws, tail, muzzle, and parts of the head. Green areas commonly encompass the neck, shoulder, side areas of the body and the base of the tail. Since preferred areas may vary between individual dogs, the "Where to pet map" should always be based on the individual preferences of the respective dog (see Fig. 24.1 for an example of the "Where to pet map" based on the preferences of my dog Balua). Accordingly, drawing such a map requires the dog owner's expertise and feedback but is usually well received and enjoyed by the children.

Children with limited or bad prior experiences with dogs, in particular, need empathic guidance but also youngsters who live with a dog in their home benefit from tutelage. The importance of having clear and mandatory instructions for recipients on how to interact with the dog cannot be overstated. Further, these instructions should be explained to the children prior to introducing the dog. Adequate pre-instructions and informed consent are particularly challenging when interventions are designed for children with psychological, developmental, and/or cognitive disabilities as these children may not fully understand or quickly forget how to behave appropriately in the presence of the dog. In such cases, close supervision and/or guidance by the DAI professional is mandatory to protect the dog. Working in small groups of children makes it easier for the DAI professional to devote the needed amount of attention to each child–dog interaction. Support from other people such as teachers or assistant volunteers can be beneficial to handle groups. In many instances, single recipient sessions may be best suited for children with a psychological, developmental, and/or cognitive disorder.

Entering School Buildings

When visiting schools and school-like environments, the human–dog dyad will usually enter a facility that accommodates a high number of people.

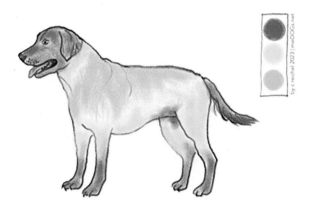

Fig. 24.1. "Where to pet map" based on the preferences of my dog Balua. Red indicates *stop* (these body parts should never be touched); yellow indicates *careful* (areas where the dog may not always enjoy being petted and increased attention on stress-related behaviors is warranted); and green indicates *OK to go* (the dog is likely to enjoy tactile contact here from most people).

Besides the importance of acquiring informed consent for a dog visit from the principal or respective authority, teachers, parents, and other staff's informed consent should be considered as well. Otherwise, a visiting therapy dog can cause irritation among caretaker or cleaning personnel, which can create additional challenges. I have experienced a case where the school caretaker asked the therapy dog owner to leave the school building with her dog immediately in an unfriendly manner, regardless of their license and special approval by the principal. Such inconvenience on either part could have been prevented if the caretaker had been informed in advance.

Additionally, the high level of noise and potential overload due to environmental stimuli that characteristically emerge during recess or playtime should be avoided. Thus, visitation dogs should enter and leave schools at a time where most children will be under supervision in their classroom. Teachers and pupils should be instructed to clean the classroom from any food leftovers prior to introduction of the dog. Accordingly, the following questions should be addressed prior to visiting a school:

- Do I have a written approval from the head of the facility?
- Has everybody directly (children, teachers, aids, etc.) or indirectly involved or affected (parents, legal representatives, principal, other staff) by the intervention been adequately informed?
- Have I inquired about the ideal time (i.e. when most children are supervised in their classroom) to enter and leave the building?

Mindful Presence and Constant Supervision

There is compelling evidence that children and adolescents cannot simply be regarded as small adults as they differ considerably in several aspects, including sensory integration of environmental stimuli, cognitive capacities, emotion regulation, impulsiveness and metabolism. Given these natural predispositions, adult supervision is mandatory in dog–child interactions to protect the animal's welfare and integrity at any time. As recent data by Bidoli *et al.* (2022) revealed, some dog handlers in their study were willing to loan their therapy dogs to colleagues or let pupils go out for a walk with the dog without any adult supervision. Inappropriate

interactions with the dog that were noted by the study authors included children grabbing, pulling or shaking the dog's ears, lips, muzzle, head, neck, tail and paws. In several cases, the dog handlers would ignore such unpleasant and risky intrusions, thereby failing to protect the dog (and the children). Not only do these behaviors significantly impact canine well-being, they can lead to withdrawal or even aggressive displays in the dogs. Thus, several implications for practice emerge:

- Each dog–child encounter must be supervised by the dog owner, who is the primary responsible person for any type of interaction.
- Each dog–child encounter must be based on mutual voluntariness.
- The dog handler must react appropriately to signs of discomfort in her or his dog. These include the more subtle stress indicators and especially refer to withdrawal behavior or attempts to escape the situation, which suggest that the dog needs more distance or time to rest.

Reducing Arousal and Promoting Calm Interactions

Children and adolescents can benefit from a wide range of interactions with dogs such as quietly reading a book to the dog, gently petting the dog, or soft play with or without toys or mild physical exercise. Both recipients and the dog may find these activities naturally exciting, which is beneficial in most cases as it raises levels of attention, focus, performance, and motivation. To maintain good health and well-being, phases of activation and arousal should be followed by periods of rest and calm. A common challenge I experience in groups is that most individuals want to make contact with the dog straight away and when they observe a classmate perform a task with the dog, they immediately raise their arm to be next and want to do the same. However, many repetitions of the same task with different recipients can be tiring for the dog. Similarly, the dog may be intimidated if approached by multiple pupils or touched by multiple hands simultaneously (see Fig. 24.2). Instead, no more than two hands at a time should be placed on the dog (see Fig. 24.3).

During phases of rest or while sleeping, the dog can be easily irritated by unwanted social

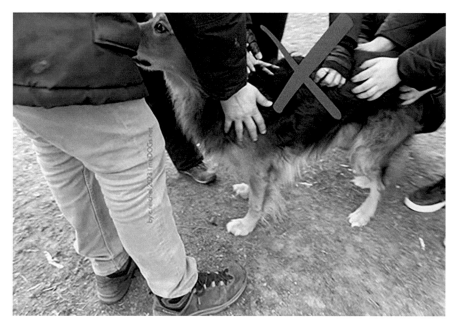

Fig. 24.2. The dog is intimidated when approached by multiple pupils and touched by multiple hands simultaneously.

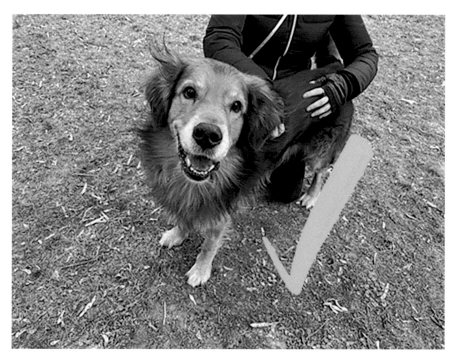

Fig. 24.3. No more than two hands at a time should be placed on the dog.

intrusions. Over the past years, research has shown that children (and many adults) fail to correctly recognize canine emotional displays (Giraudet *et al.*, 2022). Thus, they may not realize when they stress the dog's comfort zone. Accordingly, some general rules for safely interacting with the dog are helpful to support animal welfare during DAIs.

Recommendations to diversify DAIs and avoid exhaustion:

- Less is more: the dog should never be crowded by multiple recipients (see Fig. 24.2).
- As a rule, no more than two hands at a time should be touching the dog (see Fig. 24.3).
- Activities and recipients should be arranged in a way that allows the dog to withdraw at any time.
- Activities in DAIs should be adjusted to an individual dog's talent and preferences. Moreover, they should be diversified so that activating and exciting tasks are followed by quiet and calm phases.
- Establish a resting area that is exclusive to the dog (e.g. a preferred blanket, dog crate).
- Mind the level of noise in classrooms while a dog is present (children should be taught that according to differences in sensory organ function, the sensitivity to noise varies between humans and animals).

Conclusions

With the growing popularity of DAIs, ensuring superior animal welfare is now considered essential by scientists, practitioners, and leading organizations (Glenk, 2017; Glenk and Foltin, 2021). Dog handlers need to cope efficiently with challenging situations and recipients in order to protect their dog. As highlighted in this chapter, adequate preparation of the recipients, mindful guidance of human–animal interactions, and acknowledgement of the individual preferences of the therapy dog are the cornerstones of best practice DAIs.

References

Bidoli, E.M.Y., Firnkes, A., Bartels, A., Erhard, M.H. and Döring, D. (2022) Dogs working in schools–safety awareness and animal welfare. *Journal of Veterinary Behavior* 57, 35–48. DOI: 10.1016/j.jveb.2022.09.004.

Giraudet, C.S.E., Liu, K., McElligott, A.G. and Cobb, M. (2022) Are children and dogs best friends? A scoping review to explore the positive and negative effects of child-dog interactions. *PeerJ* 10, e14532. DOI: 10.7717/peerj.14532.

Glenk, L.M (2017) Current perspectives on therapy dog welfare in animal-assisted interventions. *Animals* 7(2), 7. DOI: 10.3390/ani7020007.

Glenk, L.M. and Foltin, S. (2021) Therapy dog welfare revisited: a review of the literature. *Veterinary Sciences* 8(10), 226. DOI: 10.3390/vetsci8100226.

25 Before Going Forward, Plan Backward: Prioritizing Welfare During HAIs

Terri Hlava*

Human Animal Bond In Teaching and Therapies (H.A.B.I.T.A.T.), Arizona State University, Tempe, Arizona, USA

Abstract

This chapter provides guidelines and concepts to help plan safe, effective human–animal interactions (HAIs) in school settings that prioritize and preserve the welfare of humans and other animals while also supporting instructional objectives. HAIs can positively impact socio-emotional and academic goals, but there are essential elements to consider before bringing an animal into the classroom. This chapter illustrates some of the necessary components in designing HAIs that can improve classroom climate, increase academic achievement, nurture healthy relationships, appreciate children's perspectives and lived experiences, and perhaps most importantly—maintain everyone's safety.

As you envision human–animal interaction (HAI), it's easy to get swept up in the excitement. The children will love having a dog, hamster, bird, or fish in the classroom! They'll learn science, responsibility, kindness, and empathy (Daly and Suggs, 2010; Fine and Gee, 2017). They'll be gentle with the animal and with each other. Reading fluency levels will increase (Barber and Proops, 2019). Communication skills will improve (Fine, 2015). What could possibly go wrong? And that's just the trouble—however unlikely, something may go wrong, and this chapter details a few strategies to minimize that possibility and maximize the benefits of HAI while protecting the welfare of all concerned.

Welfare is an essential element in a best practice backward plan. Prioritizing everyone's welfare begins before approaching the school principal, before obtaining parental permission for student participation, and before the children begin eagerly anticipating the arrival of their new community member or classmate. A best practice backward plan begins with the end in mind; it

evaluates possible scenarios and structures the environment and the interactions to bring about the greatest benefits and least risks for all—the animal, the children, the teacher, and the HAI practitioner. Prioritizing everyone's welfare begins at the conceptualization stage as you envision your ideal HAIs.

As you start thinking about including an animal in a classroom of grade-school (primary-school) students, some of whom have diverse abilities, similar to other experiences that you plan for your students, you want to begin by thinking about why you want to incorporate HAI into your classroom. What are the objectives? The more defined your objectives are, the better you can plan your HAIs to facilitate them. Yet even if your goals are still nebulous at this stage, safety must be the top priority—first, last, and always when working with children and animals.

Next, you want to reflect on your students to determine the animal you might want to welcome into the classroom community. Do your students

*Thlava@asu.edu

have good self-regulation skills, or are they still maturing on that dimension? Can they take turns, be gentle, change activities appropriately, or do some students have difficulty with these tasks? If some students move easily and confidently from activity to activity, consider pairing them with the students who have greater difficulty, but remember, just as it is your responsibility to monitor your students' conduct throughout the day, it is also always your responsibility to make sure that students behave appropriately when interacting with an animal at school. It's fine to have a confident student be a leader and perhaps show a timid classmate how to pet a therapy dog appropriately, for instance, so long as you don't depend on the student leader to ensure the animal's safety (or anyone else's safety).

One way to increase the likelihood that students will behave appropriately around an animal is to prepare them for these interactions. You want to involve students in conversations about the animal as soon as you've secured administrative permission to invite an animal into the classroom. Do not miss this opportunity to gain invaluable insight into your students' experiences with animals. Such discussions also give students the opportunity to ask questions and share stories about other encounters with animals. Listen carefully as these exchanges can foreshadow issues that may endanger someone's welfare. For example, although many tales will be delightful, some students may share their fears about animals. Acknowledge these feelings and remind students that a visiting animal is friendly, and in the case of a dog, well trained. Some students might mention elements of abuse or descriptions of violence involving animals. Debrief these incidents and get help for the students and families if necessary. If a student has witnessed such trauma, HAI can offer an opportunity for healing and a chance to build healthy, trusting relationships in a safe environment, but never force a student to interact with an animal. And of course, always supervise students when the animal is visiting.

Some students may not be comfortable joining the discussion, so be sure to offer other options for them to share their experiences. Remind students that they can always come to your desk and whisper their stories if they need privacy. They can draw a picture, write prose or poetry or rap, make a comic book, collage, flag, or origami art; any form of expression is preferable to none at all, because communication teaches you vital information.

If you have decided to invite a therapy dog to visit, one option, to ensure that you will have a highly qualified team, is to contact a reputable organization that conducts rigorous testing and offers team certification. The organization should also provide insurance against accidents, damage, loss, and harm. Insurance helps garner support from the school administration (and all interventions benefit from administrative support).

As you and your students continue discussing the idea of inviting a therapy dog to visit, reassure students that they will all have a chance to meet the dog, and that they can decline the opportunity if they wish. This assurance is important because it can relieve anxiety, another way to provide for someone's welfare. Perhaps students who do not want to participate can read silently or visit the school library instead. It's always a good idea to remind young students of your expectations at this point too. For example, you might tell them that everyone will remain quietly seated when the dog and handler enter the classroom. If students have any questions for the therapy dog handler, they can raise their hands, just like they do when they greet any new guests at school. These procedures, explained ahead of time, protect the dog by creating a calm and respectful environment. The handler also will appreciate this atmosphere because it will allow the dog to relax and feel comfortable easing into the visit.

Finally, taking these precautions and making these preparations will go a long way toward protecting your HAI program. These preparations will also increase the likelihood that the program will be a success. It may increase your students' motivation for reading (Noble and Holt, 2018; Rousseau and Tardif-Williams, 2019) or their reading ability (Barber and Proops, 2019; Fung, 2019; Henderson *et al.*, 2020). The program may increase attendance (O'Haire *et al.*, 2014; Barber and Proops, 2019) or help science lessons come alive. The dogs may ease some students' anxiety (Waite *et al.*, 2018; Fynn and Runacres, 2022). You might also notice some students wanting to help prepare for the dog and demonstrate increased kindness, confidence, and positive social interactions with peers (Hall *et al.*,

2016; Brelsford *et al.*, 2017). All these benefits are more likely with a backward plan in motion. With this level of planning and care, your program can be a model for other classes, helping colleagues learn how they can safely implement their own HAI programs.

Case Example I

Imagine that you've invited a registered therapy dog team to visit your third-grade classroom. Your students grow more excited as the big day nears. On Friday, Dog Day, they will meet their canine classmate for the first time! You've co-created and discussed your expectations for good behavior. The students have told you about their experiences with dogs. You've been reading dog stories in class, and the students have been learning about different dog breeds and the jobs that working dogs do. It's Thursday afternoon. The room practically buzzes with excitement, and then it happens. You notice tears streaming down the cheeks of your shiest student. He quickly hides his face behind a book as his classmates continue their conversations in great anticipation of Dog Day … .

Discussion questions

1. How do you respectfully address his distress?
2. What happens if he cannot explain his tears? How do you help him?

Case Example II

Imagine that you've invited a registered therapy dog team to visit your second-grade classroom. Your students grow more excited as the big day nears. It's finally Friday, Dog Day, and after lunch recess, they will meet their canine classmate for the first time! You've co-created and discussed your expectations for good behavior. The students have told you about their experiences with dogs. You've been reading dog stories in class, and the students have been learning about different dog breeds and the jobs that working dogs do. The room practically buzzes with excitement! While the students are at recess, the team arrives early. When the children return, they want to greet their new friends all at once.

Discussion question

1. How do you manage that excitement when the children want to rush toward the dog?

References

Barber, O. and Proops, L. (2019) Low-ability secondary school students show emotional, motivational, and performance benefits when reading to a dog versus a teacher. *Anthrozoös* 32(4), 503–518. DOI: 10.1080/08927936.2019.1621522.

Brelsford, V.L., Meints, K., Gee, N.R. and Pfeffer, K. (2017) Animal-assisted interventions in the classroom – a systematic review. *International Journal of Environmental Research and Public Health* 14(7), 669. DOI: 10.3390/ijerph14070669.

Daly, B. and Suggs, S. (2010) Teachers' experiences with humane education and animals in the elementary classroom: implications for empathy development. *Journal of Moral Education* 39(1), 101–112. DOI: 10.1080/03057240903528733.

Fine, A.H. (ed.) (2015) *Handbook on Animal-assisted Therapy: Foundations and Guidelines for Animal-assisted Interventions*, 4th edn. Academic Press, San Diego, California.

Fine, A.H. and Gee, N.R. (2017) How animals help students learn: introducing a roadmap for action. In: Gee, N.R., Fine, A.H. and McCardle, P. (eds) *How Animals Help Students Learn: Research and Practice for Educators and Mental-Health Professionals*. Routledge, Abingdon, UK, pp. 3–11. DOI: 10.4324/9781315620619.

Fung, S.C. (2019) Effect of a canine-assisted read aloud intervention on reading ability and physiological response: a pilot study. *Animals* 9(8), 474. DOI: 10.3390/ani9080474.

Fynn, W.I. and Runacres, J. (2022) Dogs at school: a quantitative analysis of parental perceptions of canine-assisted activities in schools mediated by child anxiety score and use case. *International Journal of Child Care and Education Policy* 16(1), 4. DOI: 10.1186/s40723-022-00097-x.

Hall, S.S., Gee, N.R. and Mills, D.S. (2016) Children reading to dogs: a systematic review of the literature. *PloS ONE* 11(2), e0149759. DOI: 10.1371/journal.pone.0149759.

Henderson, L., Grové, C., Lee, F., Trainer, L., Schena, H. *et al.* (2020) An evaluation of a dog-assisted reading program to support student wellbeing in primary school. *Children and Youth Services Review* 118, 105449. DOI: 10.1016/j.childyouth.2020.105449.

Noble, O. and Holt, N. (2018) A study into the impact of the reading education assistance dogs scheme on reading engagement and motivation to read among early years foundation-stage children. *Education* 46(3), 277–290. DOI: 10.1080/03004279.2016.1246587.

O'Haire, M.E., McKenzie, S.J., McCune, S. and Slaughter, V. (2014) Effects of classroom animal-assisted activities on social functioning in children with autism spectrum disorder. *The Journal of Alternative and Complementary Medicine* 20(3), 162–168. DOI: 10.1089/acm.2013.0165.

Rousseau, C.X. and Tardif-Williams, C.Y. (2019) Turning the page for Spot: the potential of therapy dogs to support reading motivation among young children. *Anthrozoös* 32(5), 665–677. DOI: 10.1080/08927936.2019.1645511.

Waite, T.C., Hamilton, L. and O'Brien, W. (2018) A meta-analysis of animal assisted interventions targeting pain, anxiety and distress in medical settings. *Complementary Therapies in Clinical Practice* 33, 49–55. DOI: 10.1016/j.ctcp.2018.07.006.

T. Hlava

26 Reading Doesn't Have To Be Ruff

JEAN KIRNAN[1]* AND ASHLEY THOMPSON[2]

[1]The College of New Jersey, Ewing Township, New Jersey, USA; [2]West Belmar Elementary School, Wall Township, New Jersey, USA

Abstract

The co-authors of this chapter have worked collaboratively for over 10 years in a dog-assisted literacy program at an elementary school. In their roles as a teacher and a dog handler, the authors are able to provide unique insights into the challenges and benefits of this school-wide program. Specifically, the chapter focuses on: (i) recruiting and selecting dog-handler teams; (ii) securing permissions and approvals; (iii) preparing students and teachers; (iv) accommodating students and dogs; and (v) managing loss.

Overview

It is Friday morning. I have awakened and I am preparing for school. I have my breakfast and walk out into the brisk morning air, excited as I prepare for the day's events. As I am walking closer to West Belmar School, I think about all of the fun ahead. I will be reading with the children. I will be comforting those in need of help who are experiencing sadness. I will be promoting social interactions. Oh look, I see my friends. They are coming over to say hello and shake my paw.

I am a therapy dog. I do many jobs in schools to help students. I wonder … who will need a friend? Who will need confidence? Who can I help keep calm and focused? Who can I soothe when someone's day is not going right?

(Bob, therapy dog)

Dogs, handlers, teachers, students, and staff are all excited when reading assistance dogs come to school. However, the dog literacy program at West Belmar Elementary School is unique in that human–dog handler teams visit every class. Typically, such programs focus on struggling readers or students new to reading. Although inclusive, the whole-school program provides unique challenges for implementation and continuance. While the introduction above is from the dog's point of view, we share our insights from the perspective of a classroom teacher (Ashley) and a dog handler (Jean).

Program Planning and Recruitment

Ashley: For several years, I had been interested in bringing a dog-assisted literacy program to my elementary school. I conducted research and wrote a district grant which was approved. In the grant I shared the goal of providing a relaxed and "dog-friendly" atmosphere, allowing students to practice the skill of reading, develop confidence and take risks as readers, build fluency, and increase socialization—all while in the presence of a non-judgmental dog.

To find volunteers I reached out to two local organizations that certify therapy dogs (Therapy Dog International and Bright & Beautiful Dogs) who in turn emailed their members about this new opportunity. Certifying organizations require that the dog and handler pass tests (sociability, obedience, and varied environments), provide liability coverage, and ensure up-to-date animal health through yearly renewals; measures which help ensure the safety and well-being of the dogs as well as the children.

I then set up interviews with my principal, the dog handlers, and the dogs. At the interview, owners shared their experiences with children and with therapy dog programs, gave references, provided their availability and grade-level preferences as well as certifications and insurances, and communicated

*Corresponding author: Jkirnan@tcnj.edu

DOI: 10.1079/9781800622616.0026

their reasons for wanting to join our program. At the end of the interview, we invited a few students down to the office to interact with the dog and owner (this gave us a good look at how the dog and owner related to children). After we conducted all the interviews, we matched each dog and handler to a classroom.

The whole-school program is challenging in recruiting and retaining enough teams. In the first year there were nine handlers, two of whom had two dogs, and three of whom visited two classrooms. Dogs ranged from terriers to Great Danes. Now in its 12th year, several of the dogs have died; and only one of the original handlers still volunteers, highlighting the difficulty in staffing a comprehensive school program.

Jean: I saw the recruitment email from my certifying organization. At the time, I only had experience visiting a senior center with my dog. I had a newly certified dog and did not know how she would react to children. I appreciated the opportunity to observe the environment and meet the students and staff that I would be working with. Prior to starting visitation, handlers should review the environment with their dog for unexpected obstacles such as parking, entryway, automatic doors, stairs, elevator, floor grating, classroom layout, and noise. Additionally, children vary greatly in their energy and movements; some dogs will do better with older children than younger children or those with impulse control issues.

Permissions and Approvals

Ashley: Students were given permission slips requiring signatures from their guardians so they had consent to participate in the program—this is repeated each year. The program was approved by the Board of Education and has been approved annually ever since. Handlers share copies of their certifications (for sociability, obedience, etc.; liability coverage; and animal health, as explained earlier) each year as they are updated.

Jean: At each visit, I ask the children if they want to pet or read to my dog. I think it is important to ensure the child has a voice in the process. Most are eager to interact, but occasionally, some are not. A child may have had a negative experience with a

dog outside of school or could just be having a bad day.

Preparing Teachers

Ashley: When the program was first launched, I gave a presentation on the expectations of the program and the goals and objectives. I gave many examples of ways therapy dogs could be utilized in the classroom which varied for the grade levels. I invited staff members who wanted to see the program in action to observe how I was implementing the program into my classroom so they could understand how to implement it themselves. When new staff members are hired the program is explained to them and they work with their grade-level partners and mentor to learn how to implement the program.

Preparing Students

Ashley: Before welcoming four-legged friends into the classroom, teachers speak to their students about their expectations and appropriate behaviors when the dogs visit. Typically, teachers will explain to their students what a therapy dog is and its purpose in their classroom: (i) to improve SEL (social emotional learning); (ii) to instill confidence in struggling readers; and (iii) to improve reading skills as they read to a non-judgmental furry friend. Teachers explain that students should always ask permission to pet the therapy dog and never get in their face. Students are reminded to be gentle and use indoor voices as some dogs are sensitive to noise or movement. On the first visit, teachers conduct a "Meet and Greet" with the furry friend and their handler (Fig. 26.1). At this time the students learn about their classroom therapy dog and their handler. Students are encouraged to ask questions so they can become familiar with these visitors who will be a regular part of their classroom.

Jean: As a handler I was most impressed with the manner in which each student at the school approached the dogs. I have worked in the kindergarten classroom since 2011 and at the start of each visit, my dog and I stop at each cluster of desks, and ask the children if they want to pet my dog. Then I go to the reading carpet with my dog and the children join in small groups formed on the basis of reading ability. A few children who

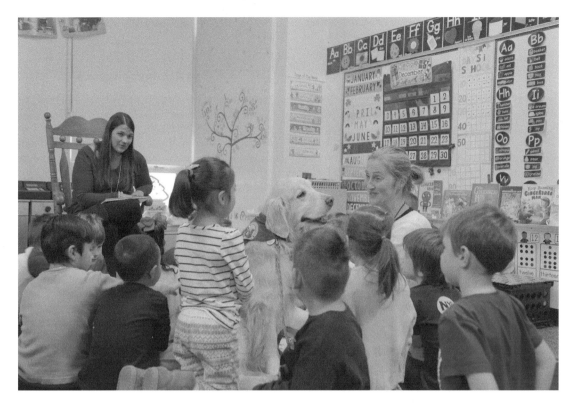

Fig. 26.1. Ashley introducing students to their therapy dog, Bob, the first day that he visited with Jean, his handler.

were afraid of the dog or unsure often sat at the furthest edge of the reading circle. However, with each weekly visit, they inched closer so that within a few months they were petting the dog and fully engaged.

Despite preparation, some children still need behavior reminders and the handler must always monitor a child's interactions with their dog. Some have impulse and self-regulation challenges and the handler must be constantly aware of a child's location and behavior as well as being attuned to the dog and their stress signs. A few students have tried to touch the dog's mouth or eyes, and one wanted to braid his tail or ear fur. While my dog would tolerate this, others would not, so I needed to gently remind everyone of the proper manner in which to pet the dog.

Even more impressive were unexpected meetings in the hallway or outside the school building. Children who knew my dog, Bob, would pass us in the hallway and want to say hello and pet him. Others didn't know him, but wanted to pet him

anyway. In either case, the children would always ask "May I pet your dog?" We'd have a brief conversation about where they were going or if they knew Bob, when they had class with him, and what grade they were in now. Even outside of the school, I would encounter children with a parent or sibling and they would approach the dog properly showing others how to do so.

Students with Accommodations

Ashley: One student had a severe allergy and was unable to read to the classroom dog. This was solved by having the student read to the dog through an iPad. Other students who are fearful of dogs remain in the classroom but at a distance. Each year that I have had a child fearful of dogs they have overcome their fears by the end and are reading to the dog. Classroom therapy dogs have also been helpful as a reward for hardworking students. Students who are struggling may work hard in the classroom to have the reward of taking a break with the dog. These students will sit and have a few quiet moments with the dog before returning to their tasks.

Jean: Another student was undergoing chemotherapy and could not attend school during regular school hours because of the risk of infection. This student would come at the end of the day to work with Ashley. The janitor sanitized the entire classroom. With parental permission, I would stay and the student would read to Bob. This created an environment of inclusion and shared activity with peers.

Dog Accommodations

Jean: Currently, my dog and I visit two kindergarten classes back to back. Scheduling needs to ensure the dog is not overworked. Most professional guidelines suggest a 15-min break after 1.5 hours; but this depends on the environment. Noise level, number of children, activity level, proximity to the dog, and type of interaction may warrant a shorter time

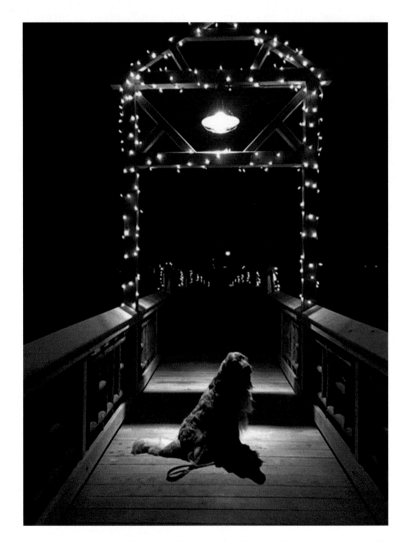

Fig. 26.2. A well-known poem, the "Rainbow Bridge" (Anon., nd), offers comfort when a pet dies. The loss of a therapy dog must be handled with compassion and empathy.

J. Kirnan and A. Thompson

frame. Handlers must be able to read their animal and observe signs of fatigue or stress. Additionally, in a school setting, handlers need to be prepared for fire drills, active shooter drills, or dismissal bells. The sound of the alarms may be frightening for your dog. It's important for the handler to know where to go and what to do in the event of a drill or an actual emergency.

Saying Goodbye—Retirement and Loss

Jean: Some organizations require retesting of the dog every 2–3 years which can help in making the decision to retire a dog. Regardless, you as the handler should consider if your dog is still able and is still enjoying the work. For handlers who spend many years at a school, it can be difficult when a dog dies. Consideration of retirement can often ease this process but not always. An unexpected death needs to be dealt with carefully considering the level of understanding of the children (Fig. 26.2). Working with the classroom teacher and a school counselor can turn this loss into a valuable learning opportunity.

Case Example I

"I'll bring my dog in next week. He loves children!" I've heard from teachers at other schools that after an animal-assisted intervention (AAI) program has begun, colleagues often assume that any dog is now welcome in the classroom.

Discussion question

1. What are the concerns if an uncertified, uninsured dog visits at school? Consider the impact that a negative incident would have not only on the dog, their owner, and the children, but also the broader AAI program.

Case Example II

At West Belmar Elementary School most of the classroom teachers enjoy the reading program. However, over the years, a small percentage of staff members have been reluctant to participate in the program. Their reasoning was typically that they didn't have time.

Discussion question

1. What can be done to encourage staff to participate in dog-assisted reading programs?

Reference

Anon (n.d.) Rainbow bridge. Available at: https://www.rainbowsbridge.com/Poem.htm (accessed 8 August 2023).

27 Canine-assisted Educational Activities in a University Setting: Reflecting on Ways to Promote Happy and Mutually Beneficial Experiences

HELEN LEWIS*

Swansea University, Swansea, UK

Abstract

This chapter outlines how canine-assisted educational (CAE) activities are undertaken with students in one university setting. Preconditions and pedagogical principles considered essential for happy, healthy human–canine interactions are discussed. The impact of these are explored through practical examples and reflections.

Swansea University is based in south Wales, UK. The canine-assisted educational (CAE) activities explored in this chapter take place in the Department of Education and Childhood Studies. Since many students in the department will go on to work as teachers or in other educational contexts, they need to become aware not only of the potential benefits of involving dogs in education, but how to do this effectively, and when it may not be appropriate. To this end, I teach a module within the BA (Hons) education degree called "An Introduction to Educational Anthrozoology". The module aims to:

- inform students of the nature and the significance of the human–animal bond;
- encourage students to evaluate the potential positive and negative impacts of animal-assisted educational approaches and identify key practical considerations; and
- allow students the opportunity to explore moral and ethical issues in relation to animal-assisted education, including animal welfare.

We also run sessions on health and well-being for postgraduate student teachers where animal-assisted interventions are explored, and sessions on animal-assisted play therapy for Master's students studying therapeutic play. All these students have opportunities to reframe how they think about the interactions between animals and children, with an emphasis on the agency of non-human animals, particularly dogs. I am assisted by my three dogs, Carlo, Scarlet, and Obie who attend sessions at various points during the semester. Each dog has a different personality and I ensure that I match the dog to the type of session and the student group (Table 27.1).

The model that underpins all elements of the sessions within this module is based upon four preconditions and four pedagogical principles (Lewis and Grigg, forthcoming; Lewis and Grigg, 2022), designed to promote the well-being of all involved (Table 27.2).

At the start of the module, all preconditions are considered, discussed with students and colleagues, and met (Table 27.3).

---

*Helen.e.lewis@swansea.ac.uk

© CAB International 2024. *Animal-assisted Interventions: Recognizing and Mitigating Potential Welfare Challenges* (ed. L.R. Kogan)
DOI: 10.1079/9781800622616.0027

Table 27.1. Carlo, Scarlet, and Obie "Getting to Know You".

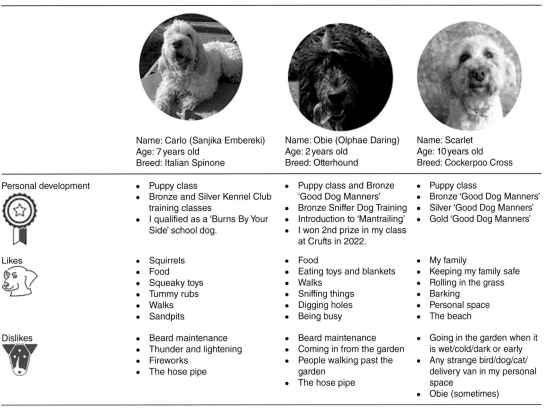

	Name: Carlo (Sanjika Embereki) Age: 7 years old Breed: Italian Spinone	Name: Obie (Olphae Daring) Age: 2 years old Breed: Otterhound	Name: Scarlet Age: 10 years old Breed: Cockerpoo Cross
Personal development	• Puppy class • Bronze and Silver Kennel Club training classes • I qualified as a 'Burns By Your Side' school dog.	• Puppy class and Bronze 'Good Dog Manners' • Bronze Sniffer Dog Training • Introduction to 'Mantrailing' • I won 2nd prize in my class at Crufts in 2022.	• Puppy class • Bronze 'Good Dog Manners' • Silver 'Good Dog Manners' • Gold 'Good Dog Manners'
Likes	• Squirrels • Food • Squeaky toys • Tummy rubs • Walks • Sandpits	• Food • Eating toys and blankets • Walks • Sniffing things • Digging holes • Being busy	• My family • Keeping my family safe • Rolling in the grass • Barking • Personal space • The beach
Dislikes	• Beard maintenance • Thunder and lightening • Fireworks • The hose pipe	• Beard maintenance • Coming in from the garden • People walking past the garden • The hose pipe	• Going in the garden when it is wet/cold/dark or early • Any strange bird/dog/cat/delivery van in my personal space • Obie (sometimes)

Given the scope of this chapter, one precondition, related to the importance of developing an understanding of canine communication and how this is met, is discussed.

Precondition 1—Canine Communication

We introduce canine communication with the use of social-media images. Social media is full of images of dogs and people interacting. Oftentimes these are heart-warming pictures, but there are some images which show dogs in difficult situations such as being hugged, kissed, or jumped upon. We take time to explore what these images tell us about canine communication and why these situations may be undesirable. For example, Fig. 27.1 is adapted from a photograph on social media.

Without knowing the individual dog (and acknowledging a photograph is a snapshot in time) it is impossible to know whether this was a comfortable interaction for her. However, we found images like these useful to open debate and awareness. As a class we identify some potential concerns. First, the dog is surrounded by several children, who are gathered closely around her. Many dogs would find this overwhelming. The dog has no easy escape route, her body looks tense, her ears are back, and her forehead is furrowed. She is looking away from the children towards the photographer, which may be a sign that she needs reassurance, is feeling stressed or anxious. We identify several ways the interaction could be improved. For example, the number of children and the nature of their interaction should be carefully managed, and the dog should be able to leave the activity at any point.

Pedagogical Principles

Having considered (and met) the necessary preconditions, we next turn to four key pedagogical principles used to guide the CAE experiences (Lewis and Grigg, 2022). These help ensure healthy, happy

Table 27.2. A model of practice for happy, humane interactions.

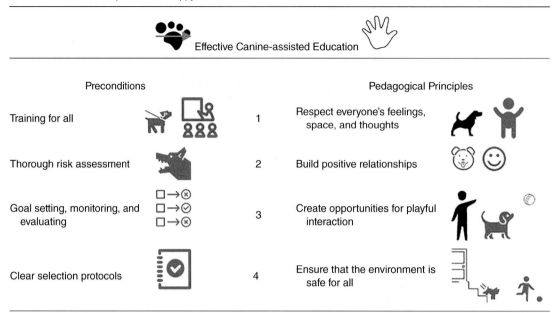

Table 27.3. Model of practice: preconditions and examples of how these are met.

Preconditions[a]	Examples
1. Develop student understanding of canine communication and the language of AAI in general	• Teach students how to observe a dog's natural behavior, "read" their signs, and respond appropriately • Ensure animals are not objectified (e.g. they are introduced as individuals, not "it", and are *involved* not "used" in sessions) • Explore how to meet and greet a dog, how to stroke, and how to ask for consent to interact with them
2. Ensure risk assessment is robust and considers all participants	• Identify hazards with students (e.g. accidental injury, damage caused to university property, hygiene, allergies, phobias, and cultural/religious considerations) • Consider how to eliminate/reduce risks (e.g. supervision, communication, training) • Ensure risks to dogs are identified and mitigated against (e.g. unfamiliar spaces and people, travel) • Prepare for the unexpected (e.g. fire alarms, weather)
3. Ensure the intervention is clearly planned (e.g. to impact student's learning or well-being, and dog's well-being)	• Identify sound pedagogical reasons for bringing dogs into sessions • Employ a clear rationale to select the individual dog best suited to the activities • Consider how the dog will benefit (e.g. when playing a game with a favorite soft toy)
4. Establish clear selection protocols for students, dogs, and handlers	• Match the right dog with the right student, and in the right environment • Acknowledge all participants are individuals • Allow participants choices about when and with whom they interact • Observe participants throughout the session as an ongoing process

[a]AAI, animal-assisted intervention.

H. Lewis

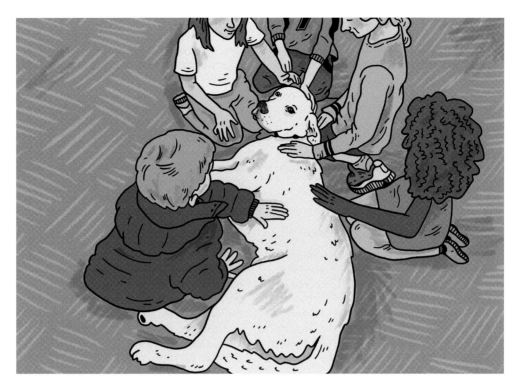

Fig. 27.1. Surrounding the dog.

and humane interactions for both the students and the dogs.

1. Respect everyone's feelings, spaces, and thoughts

Carlo, Scarlet, and Obie do not have a choice in whether they are present in the university on a specific day, but they do have agency over whether they wish to interact with students. They can indicate their consent in several non-verbal ways. The students need to get to know each dog as an individual and observe their behaviour throughout the interaction to ensure they are willing participants. My role is to have a plan in place if the dog indicates that they do not want to join in.

2. Build positive relationships

Successful relationships are based on values such as care, kindness, and connection, and take time to develop (Van Fleet and Faa-Thompson, 2017).

Just like people, dogs will have preferred friends, and just like us, dogs do not love unconditionally (Bekoff, 2019). Expectations around the dogs need to be discussed and carefully managed. If a dog chooses not to interact with a particular student, for instance, this may have detrimental effects on their well-being.

3. Create opportunities for playful interaction

Dogs enjoy playing, so it is important that interactions are based on playful learning. This does not mean that dogs should be regarded as playthings, rather as play partners. Playful learning also benefits dogs, because it helps their mental health and enables the formation of strong bonds (Van Fleet and Faa-Thompson, 2017).

4. Ensure that the environment is safe for all

The university is very different from Carlo, Scarlet, and Obie's home environment. It is vital that we know and understand the dog as fully as we can, so that we can predict the things that they will delight in and anticipate the things that may cause them stress. There also need to be clear guidelines regarding the dog's right to a quiet space to retreat to, where they can rest and relax.

Clear communication with students and careful risk assessment are also essential. Appropriate health and safety measures need to be in place to minimize harm to all participants. For example, some students may be afraid or allergic to dogs. These situations must be handled appropriately to ensure everyone's well-being.

Bringing the Principles Together

The Animal Assisted Intervention International (2019) Standards of Practice emphasize that the dog needs to be able to rely on their human partner. This means that emotional and physical support is in place for the dog. The university is different from home in terms of the sensory environment dogs experience. Glenk and Foltin (2021) suggest that dogs need time to explore

a novel setting. Therefore, before any session involving the dogs, I consider the support they need to thrive. We get to the room in advance of the students, and the dog has time off the lead to explore. I bring familiar bedding, bowls, and toys (Principles 1 and 4). Once students arrive, they are encouraged to watch each dog to observe their body language and behaviour, which we then discuss.

Students also observe the dogs around the campus to identify places where they may feel anxious or unsure, and to consider how to mitigate against this (Principles 1, 2, and 4). The students then record and discuss what they notice, and analyse what they feel; this tells them about how the dog might be feeling (Table 27.4).

We also use videos to explore canine body language (Principles 1, 2, and 4). For example, we might watch how Obie approaches the electronic entrance doors. Being able to replay the video offers the opportunity to improve reflections because students can view each clip several times. In one video, Obie appeared anxious in the elevator. We discussed an action plan for how we could support

Table 27.4. Student observations of Obie moving around campus.

Location	Why was this selected?	Student observations
Stairs	Obie does not go upstairs at home	Relaxed and inquisitive Interested in treats Looked at Helen and waited behind her until she moved He followed calmly
Main entrance	Electric doors may move or sound frightening	Obie watched people enter Didn't react to sound or movement of doors Sniffed ground in relaxed manner Made eye contact with Helen before moving through calmly when he was ready
Narrow first-floor corridor with slippery floor	Small space, unfamiliar texture and quite echoey	Obie focused on Helen who spoke to him as they walked
Metal drain covers in grounds	Sound and feel unfamiliar	Avoided at first Sniffed around with relaxed body language Stopped to watch a seagull Stepped onto cover confidently to get a treat when he was ready
Elevator	Brand new experience, loud, small space, movement	Relaxed when entering Body tensed as doors closed When doors opened left rapidly, tail tucked

H. Lewis

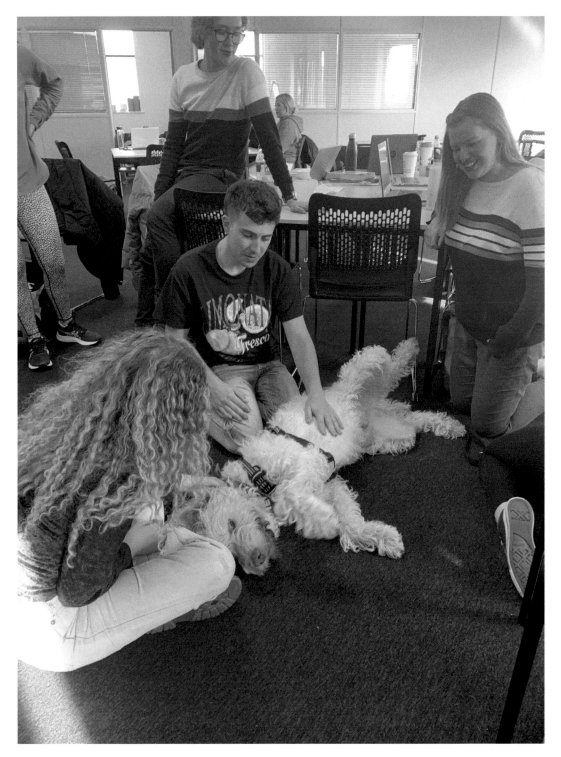

Fig. 27.2. Carlo being petted by the student teachers.

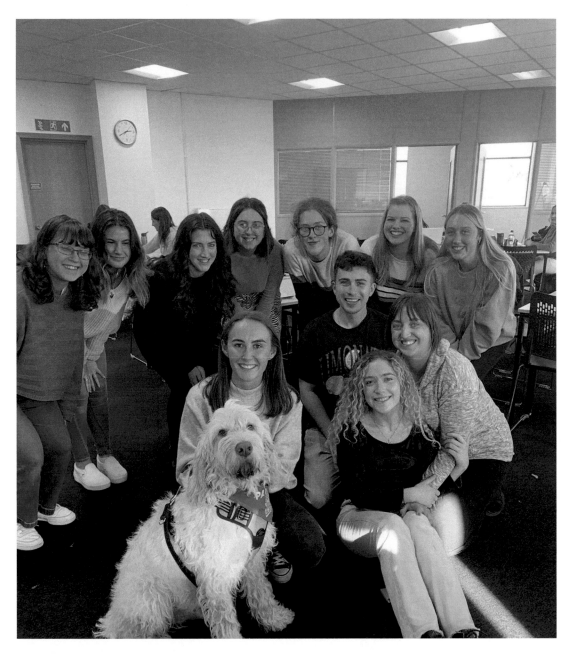

Fig. 27.3. Carlo and the student teachers.

him to feel more confident—or whether using the stairs was actually a better option.

Once we have explored canine communication, students are asked to re-create the social-media image, but make it better to demonstrate their own understanding of happy, healthy interactions (Principles 1, 2, and 4).

In Fig. 27.2 Carlo is not crowded or pressured, the students are a respectful distance from him, and have asked his consent to be stroked. He has options should he wish to leave. His body language suggests he is relaxed. Once he did move, he was allowed to walk around the class, before being invited back. He came to the group of students, who again avoided crowding him while taking a group picture (Fig. 27.3).

Immediately after this photo he had the chance to play "fetch" with his stuffed squirrel (Principle 3). His love of his toy meant that he was keen to play games such as "Find It" with the students, and his excitement was shared by the group.

My Role

There are numerous considerations that I make. For example, my dogs do not come to sessions every week. They come regularly enough for the experience to be familiar, but still engaging for them and the students. They do not stay all day, and regular rest periods are scheduled. The dogs remain my responsibility while they are on campus. I do not bring them to work in the heat of summer, because the car journey is 40 min, and the campus is not fully air conditioned. I bring one dog into my class at a time, because I can only fully focus on one. If the sessions would benefit from the input of more than one dog, a member of my family comes to assist with handling. If at any point the dog indicates that they are unsettled or uncomfortable, the session is paused and they are taken to their safe space.

This is hard work. However, the dogs themselves behave in a relaxed, engaged manner, and I believe the experiences enrich their lives. Student feedback is positive, attendance and engagement is high, and hopefully the next generation of educators will better understand the potential of animal-assisted activities—and ways to develop these that ensure the welfare of all involved.

Acknowledgement

Thank you to Russell Grigg and Tom Bradraw for bringing the figures and tables to life.

Bibliography

Animal Assisted Intervention International (2019) Standards of practice. Available at: https://aai-int.org/aai/standards-of-practice/ (accessed 17 March 2023).

Bekoff, M. (2019) Dogs watch us carefully and read our faces very well. *Psychology Today* 13 April. Available at: https://www.psychologytoday.com/gb/blog/animal-emotions/201904/dogs-watch-us-carefully-and-read-our-faces-very-well (accessed 18 March 2023).

Glenk, L.M. and Foltin, S. (2021) Therapy dog welfare revisited: a review of the literature. *Veterinary Sciences* 8(10), 226. DOI: 10.3390/vetsci8100226.

Lewis, H. and Grigg, R. (forthcoming) *Taking the Lead: Pedagogy and Practice for Happy, Healthy and Humane School Dog Interventions*. Routledge, Abingdon, UK.

Lewis, H. and Grigg, R. (2022) *Tails from the Classroom: Learning and Teaching Through Animal-assisted Interventions*. Crown House, Carmarthen, UK.

Lewis, H., Grigg, R. and Knight, C. (2022) An international survey of animals in schools: exploring what sorts of schools involve what sorts of animals, and educators' rationales for these practices. *People and Animals: The International Journal of Research and Practice* 5(1), Article 15. Available at: https://docs.lib.purdue.edu/paij/vol5/iss1/15 (accessed 17 March 2023).

McConnell, P.B. (2002) *The Other End of the Leash: Why We Do What We Do Around Dogs*. Ballantine Books, New York.

Swansea University (2023) *EDN209 Module Handbook*. Swansea University, Swansea, UK.

Van Fleet, R. and Faa-Thompson, T. (2017) *Animal Assisted Play Therapy*. Professional Resource Press.

28 Enhancing Dog–Human Communication in Animal-assisted Programs

Kirsty MacQueen*

Therapawsitive CIC, Glasgow, Scotland, UK

Abstract

Observing animals on an ongoing basis—to ensure their emotional well-being is continuously assessed—interpreting and responding (when needed) requires a strong understanding of dog behavior and communication, in conjunction with the circumstances and environments which allow this clear dialogue to occur. Canine communication provides a valuable tool to assess the emotional comfort of dogs. By maximizing both the dogs' ability to communicate and the practitioners' ability to capture that information—as a deliberate feature of animal-assisted intervention (AAI) program design—one can deliver interactions which enhance the quality, welfare, and safety, for both dogs and people.

While it is important for therapists and practitioners to make sure their animals are not displaying stress signals, that is not enough. We want animals who are eager to be there, who initiate interactions, who display signs of enjoyment, and who freely make choices of their own about the activities, their participation, and their interactions with people.

(Dr. Risë VanFleet, Boiling Springs, Pennsylvania, February 7, 2023, personal communication)

It is widely accepted that observations of animal behavior can help us interpret internal states (Fraser, 2009) and give us a window into the animal's experience. Observations in animal-assisted intervention (AAI) often depend strongly on the ability to split attention between our animal and human participant(s). Even seasoned ethologists and dog behavior consultants—having spent countless hours studying behaviors and observing animals in a focused way—may find the realities of splitting attention and conducting observations, in some of the diverse AAI settings, a challenge. Dogs are able to demonstrate a flexible repertoire of interspecific communication with humans (Siniscalchi *et al.*, 2018; Wynne, 2019), including but not limited

to, a range of visual and vocal communication (Siniscalchi *et al.*, 2018), attention-getting behaviors, referential behaviors—which intentionally direct another's attention towards a target (Worsley and O'Hara, 2018)—and play signals (Horowitz and Bekoff, 2007). Acquiring a professional level of skill to attentively observe, accurately interpret, and appropriately respond to this wide range of canine behavior should therefore be a priority component in the training, assessment, and certification for all practitioners of animal-assisted programs.

The ability to accurately interpret and respond to this wide range of canine communication may play an important role in the development of the AAI dog's behavioral vocabulary, giving them confidence to calmly and safely indicate "no thanks" and "yes please" in a variety of contexts, which can further aide understanding of their experience of these interactions. Is a dog that will stand and tolerate an interaction they do not enjoy, such as a child hugging tightly around their neck, preferable to a dog that would calmly move from that child to prevent being hugged (enthusiastically returning when the child

---

*Kirstykmq@gmail.com

© CAB International 2024. *Animal-assisted Interventions: Recognizing and Mitigating Potential Welfare Challenges* (ed. L.R. Kogan)
DOI: 10.1079/9781800622616.0028

adjusts their behavior)? A dog that is empowered with calm, safe, and confident communication skills, and the circumstances which allow their use, has the ability to exert some control over their own well-being and their enjoyment of interactions. When a dog has a strong history of working with people who observe, *listen*, and offer alternative choices which are fun, interesting, aligned with the dog's own preferences, they may feel empowered to request those alternatives instead of merely tolerating those which are not so enjoyable.

To facilitate and encourage this canine communication there are a number of adaptations that can be incorporated into program design, many of which were developed by implementing the Animal Assisted Play Therapy™ (VanFleet and Faa-Thompson, 2017) framework to that process. These are:

- *Preparation*: introductory sessions (with no dog present) for participants to learn about dog communication and the preferences of the individual dog they will work with.
- *People*: only one person interacting with the dog at any one time (especially when petting) to give the dog the freedom to move away, and the ability to have a conversation with that individual.
- *Place*: working in open space (not surrounded by furniture or people) to allow the dog to use their full body to communicate, without restricting their movement.
- *Proximity*: working mainly off-leash (where it is safe to do so) giving the dog freedom to increase and decrease proximity from interactions as desired.
- *Playfulness*: including activities which are playful and include the dog as an active participant permits observation of willingness to engage and enjoy the activity. Avoiding activities where the dog is a prop (being used, but not truly included in the activity) and those which require the dog to remain stationary, which may suppress natural behavior and communication, and inhibit expression of their emotional experience.
- *Pause*: regular opportunities for breaks within sessions to see if there is voluntary re-engagement and enthusiasm to return to activities and interactions.
- *Privacy*: a dedicated *people-free* zone (referred to as the *"safe zone"* in Animal Assisted Play Therapy™ policies (VanFleet, 2023)) and as

space which "children and participants are not permitted to invade" as recommended in the LEAD Risk Assessment Tool best practice standards (Brelsford *et al.*, 2020, p. 7) where the dog can clearly indicate a need to rest or end an interaction without being followed.

Facilitating these contexts, which enhance the dog's choice and ability to communicate, also increases the available information to evaluate their emotional well-being. Through a continuous observational process (shown in Fig. 28.1) it is possible to create a *live* risk assessment of the emotional well-being of dogs involved in AAI, thereby identifying opportunities to respond and improve well-being when it is suboptimal. Responses may range from a short interrupt or redirect of client's behavior, a change of activity, or the need to remove the dog and end the session early. A frequent requirement to respond to support the animal may also highlight that something in the session is not working as anticipated (prompting a re-evaluation of compatibility of dog, human, and/or program design). By checking continuously for indicators that the animal is not merely tolerating the interaction or showing signs (which may be subtle) of discomfort or stress, and actively noting the presence of behaviors which indicate positive affect, it is possible to improve the welfare of the animal (Boissy *et al.*, 2007).

All of the adaptations outlined, utilized in combination, support the dog's ability to communicate and the practitioner's ability to use that information to assess dog well-being and respond to improve it. There is still much to learn about dog–human communication, so by acknowledging the strengths and limitations of our dog communication knowledge (in research and in our individual practice) we can continue to reflect, to develop, and combine ideas, which can improve the emotional well-being of animals involved in AAI. Developments in our understanding of, and utilization of, dog–human and human–dog communication is one of the most powerful tools available to enhance the well-being and safety of our animals, and the people we support.

Case Example I

Bug does not mind being patted on the head, but like many dogs he does not *enjoy* it. On one occasion a caretaker supporting a child reached out—as many people naturally do—to pet Bug on the head. When

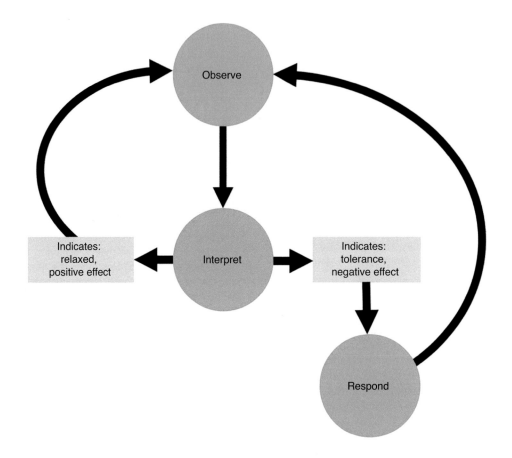

Fig. 28.1. Observe, interpret and respond: continuous assessment of dog behavior and communication to evaluate canine emotional well-being in animal-assisted interventions. Dynamic interactions between people and dogs require ongoing observation to ensure well-being and safety for all participants.

Bug side stepped slightly out of reach and waited for the adult to adjust his behavior and try again, the young person said "remember, not his head". Again, this adult reached for Bug's head. Before I was able to intervene and advocate, Bug did a little exaggerated bounce, just out of reach, turned around and reversed; walking backwards to point his rear end towards the man's feet. Here he waited. After a few seconds of confusion the caretaker realized what Bug's request was and complied by petting him on his lower back, just above the tail (exactly where he likes most!). The young person responded by stating "that means Bug trained you now", which brought laughs from all. The child's caretaker had been present in the introductory session where Bug's preferred "petting zones" were explained and yet it was Bug's ability to communicate "no thanks" and indicate "this instead please" which impacted the caretaker's actions and created an interaction which they could both enjoy. Bug was able to demonstrate agency in a way that ended one human behavior and initiated another. Though advocacy was available from both the child and myself, ultimately this was not required.

Discussion questions

1. How can we encourage dogs to further develop agency, and use these calm and confident communication skills with people?
2. How might this scenario be different, from the dog's perspective, if he was on a leash or the environment placed restrictions on his freedom of movement?

K. MacQueen

Case Example II

Working with a small group of young teenagers who were not attending mainstream classes, we carefully co-designed an activity which would involve carrying out a risk assessment of the school grounds, taking a dog's-eye perspective, so that scented objects could be hidden in safe places for the dog to search and find. I requested the school provide a staff member to assist for the duration of the program. This staff member was responsible for the teens, so that my priority focus could always be on observing and advocating for my dog. Part way through the activity, two of the teenagers started to play in a physical way that I recognized was likely to spill over into an altercation. The teens were made aware at the start of the program if any of their behavior might be unsafe for the dog (who could accidentally be caught in the crossfire) that we would immediately leave and return only if/when they were behaving in a safe way. With the second adult available, I was easily able to do that immediately. As we left, the other teenagers could be heard telling the two boys that Bug (my dog) was leaving. That prompted them to stop, apologize to each other, and then ask if they could come and apologize to Bug.

Discussion questions

1. When working with groups, especially in environments that—even with the most careful planning—can remain somewhat unpredictable (e.g. schools, prison, community settings), is it possible to split attention and provide sufficient observation of the dog and multiple children without at least one additional adult?
2. How do you feel modeling behaviors that reflect the importance of dog safety and emotional well-being can impact your relationship with a client or participant?

Bibliography

Boissy, A., Manteuffel, G., Jensen, M.B., Moe, R.O., Spruijt, B. *et al.* (2007) Assessment of positive emotions in animals to improve their welfare. *Physiology & Behavior* 92(3), 375–397. DOI: 10.1016/j.physbeh.2007.02.003.

Brelsford, V.L., Dimolareva, M., Gee, N.R. and Meints, K. (2020) Best practice standards in animal-assisted interventions: how the LEAD risk assessment tool can help. *Animals* 10(6), 974. DOI: 10.3390/ani10060974.

Fraser, D. (2009) Animal behaviour, animal welfare and the scientific study of affect. *Applied Animal Behaviour Science* 118(3–4), 108–117. DOI: 10.1016/j.applanim.2009.02.020.

Horowitz, A.C. and Bekoff, M. (2007) Naturalizing anthropomorphism: behavioral prompts to our humanizing of animals. *Anthrozoös* 20(1), 23–35. DOI: 10.2752/089279307780216650.

Serpell, J.A., Coppinger, R., Fine, A.H. and Peralta, J.M. (2010) Welfare considerations in therapy and assistance animals. In: Fine, A.H. (ed.) *Handbook on Animal-Assisted Therapy: Theoretical Foundations and Guidelines for Practice*, 3rd edn. Academic Press, Cambridge, Massachusetts, pp. 481–503. DOI: 10.1016/B978-0-12-381453-1.10023-6.

Siniscalchi, M., d'Ingeo, S., Minunno, M. and Quaranta, A. (2018) Communication in dogs. *Animals* 8(8), 131. DOI: 10.3390/ani8080131.

VanFleet, R. (2023) Animal assisted play therapy. Available at: https://risevanfleet.com/aapt/ (accessed 8 August 2023).

VanFleet, R. and Faa-Thompson, T. (2017) *Animal Assisted Play Therapy*. Professional Resource Press, Sarasota, Florida.

Worsley, H.K. and O'Hara, S.J. (2018) Cross-species referential signalling events in domestic dogs (*Canis familiaris*). *Animal Cognition* 21(4), 457–465. DOI: 10.1007/s10071-018-1181-3.

Wynne, C.D. (2019) *Dog Is Love: Why and How Your Dog Loves You*. Houghton Mifflin Harcourt, Boston, Massachusetts.

29 Welfare and Safety Considerations in AAI Hospital Programs

CYNNIE FOSS*

University of Washington Medical Center, Seattle, Washington, USA

Abstract

With the growing popularity, acceptance, and proven benefits of animal-assisted interventions (AAIs) in hospitals, it has become increasingly important to educate teams, staff, and participants that animal welfare is essential to the success and sustainability of AAI programs. This chapter seeks to examine the importance of prioritizing training, recognition, and mitigation of any potential welfare red flags in the animal or in the AAI setting.

There is no doubt that animal-assisted interventions (AAIs) bring immense joy in a hospital setting for both patients and staff. For patients, an AAI intervention can lead to lower heart rate, reduced blood pressure, stress relief, sense of calm, and comfort in an otherwise sterile environment. When surveyed, staff at my medical center have indicated that an intervention decreases their own stress levels, increases job satisfaction, elevates mood, provides needed tactile interaction, creates a sense of community, and provides comfort. What often is not perceived by those involved with this type of interaction is the importance of: (i) animal- (referred to as "dog" moving forward) team training/credentialing; (ii) team screening (animal, handler, and guide for fit); (iii) action planning for variable outcomes; and (iv) the need for continual observation to ensure a safe visit for the patient/ staff member, but also the dog and handler. Even the best-trained therapy dog can have visits where something is off: they may show signs of being tired or disinterested, or the environment is too chaotic, or patients or staff do not interact appropriately, etc. Any of these can lead to a visible behavior that warrants a mitigating response by the handler and AAI staff or volunteer guide. Depending on the situation the appropriate action can be ending a session altogether.

There are only a small handful of legitimate non-profit agencies that evaluate pet therapy or AAI teams. Unfortunately, the rating system of teams that pass these practical tests is not standardized across agencies. Additionally, there is no evaluating agency follow-up with teams on site at the organizations where they volunteer. While many of these practical tests are quite stringent, they do not evaluate if the handler and dog are a suitable fit for a specific hospital environment. Ultimately, this is up to the staff AAI coordinator on site and the registered handler. In a hospital setting, it is important to determine if the therapy team is appropriate for patients or staff only; not every team is a good fit for both. Therefore, creating a standard for both settings (e.g. patient and staff) is the first step to ensuring the welfare of the dog by setting them up for success in an appropriate environment that suits their personality and ability. The staff coordinator must determine if the handler is interested and able to work well with extremely ill patients and spend time with the dog to see if they are suited to quiet one-on-one meetings. Additionally, it is equally important to recognize that working with staff typically involves loud group settings. Ideally, the staff coordinator is trained to understand the basics of AAIs and has practical experience of their own. I was a pet therapy team with my dog for

*Fossc@uw.edu

© CAB International 2024. *Animal-assisted Interventions: Recognizing and Mitigating Potential Welfare Challenges* (ed. L.R. Kogan)
DOI: 10.1079/9781800622616.0029

3 years, I manage the pet therapy program for two large city hospitals and have earned a certificate in "Dog Behavior and Training for Provider of Animal-Assisted Intervention" from the Center for Human Animal Intervention at Oakland University, Michigan. All this background has given me invaluable insight in selecting teams for different interactions.

In addition to the teams, it is necessary to have a staff or volunteer guide present for every AAI interaction. This guide must understand how vital their role is and what constitutes a successful visit for the participants and the team. While the handler should be focused on their dog's welfare throughout, the guide should be more focused on the participants, yet also helping to observe the dog's behavior. Pet Partners refers to this as YAYABA—"You are your animal's best advocate". Being the best advocate means understanding and recognizing animal behavior that might be unfavorable to continued participation. A handler knows their dog better than anyone else. However, it is quite easy to get caught up in the moment of talking with a patient or staff member and not realize that there is a growing welfare-related situation. Juggling the leash of the dog, interacting with participants, answering questions, ensuring participants are following strict hand hygiene—it can be quite overwhelming for the handler, not to mention the dog. Constant monitoring is important and a two-person system (e.g. handler and guide) is recommended. The handler and the guide should remain within talking distance so they can communicate effectively and there should be a determined action plan should the dog show any behavior or physical signs of distress.

This chapter addresses the importance of animal welfare in AAI visits and the significance of experienced staff and teams, training, and education to ensure a safe environment for all. AAI in a hospital setting is more complex than other settings, but with proper management, comprehensive training, and consistent stewardship of the involved teams, it can and will be successful, bringing needed joy and comfort to those it benefits.

Case Example I

An experienced AAI team was unexpectedly stationed in a nursing unit elevator lobby due to the regular meeting space being unavailable. All seemed fine at first, but then both the handler and the guide observed the dog backing away from staff participants. This normally sociable, friendly, loving dog was staying close to his handler and not walking out from her to greet staff who wanted to pet him. I noticed him circling a couple times, then sitting, then looking at his handler. We discussed the situation after a group left and soon realized that the dog was reacting to the intermittent dinging of the elevator stopping on the floor. The sound combined with the constant opening and closing of the elevator seemed to be causing the reaction. The handler was upset because she had never seen her dog react this way.

Discussion question

1. What might the handler or guide do at this point to mitigate potential welfare concerns?

Case Example II

In this case scenario, there was a very experienced AAI team partnered with a new guide who had no previous AAI training. The guide was a former employee and subsequently started conversing with all the staff she knew. As a result, she was distracted and out of ear shot of the handler. During the visit, a staff person started repeatedly running up behind the dog and touching the dog from behind and then running away—as if she were afraid of the dog but wanted to try and touch it. The handler noticed this was causing the dog anxiety and distraction (the dog was turning around, not engaging with the people in front due to this distraction). The handler tried to tell this person to stop what she was doing but the person was not receptive. The result was that both the dog and the handler became quite anxious, and the handler had to stop the session to ensure that her dog was OK. This was very upsetting for the handler and the staff who were excited to interact with the dog.

Discussion question

1. What could the handler and guide have done differently to lead to a different result?

30 A Humane Education Journey: Teaching and Learning Compassion

URSULA A. ARAGUNDE KOHL*

Universidad Ana G. Méndez, Gurabo Campus, Gurabo, Puerto Rico

Abstract

This chapter describes how therapy dogs can help instructors teach about humane education. This approach not only serves to educate the community but also to showcase the benefits of animal companionship. Through activities and storytelling, instructors partnering with therapy dogs can foster compassion, action, and critical thinking, helping participants understand the interconnectedness of people and animals and how they can become part of the solution.

Since 2010, one of my primary goals has been to educate individuals on our communities' needs, responsibilities, and opportunities regarding animal welfare, particularly companion animals that reside on the streets of Puerto Rico. To accomplish this goal, I have used my resources at the University Ana G. Méndez, Gurabo Campus and the non-profit Puerto Rico Alliance for Companion Animals, Inc. (PR Animals) (available at: www.pranimals.org (accessed February 12 2023)) and employed my two certified therapy dogs. Both are rescued and exemplify what we can achieve when cultivating a culture of compassion, responsibility, and inclusion. I firmly believe that most experts in this field would agree that companion animals visiting schools, universities, and community centers can be a very effective way to teach and attract attention to the importance of human–animal interactions. This approach educates the community and showcases the benefits of animal companionship, which can improve mental and physical health.

When choosing therapy dogs, I consider several factors, including temperament, enthusiasm, and energy level. Working in animal welfare has allowed me to foster and rehabilitate numerous dogs and gain experience with different breeds and personalities. With this privilege comes the ability to accurately identify dogs suitable for this type of work. The most critical attribute is the desire to interact with people, particularly strangers. This concept is vital. Even loving guardians of "perfect" dogs may struggle to understand that their dogs may only tolerate interactions with strangers and not necessarily enjoy them. As dog owners, we often want to share our pets with others, but it is essential to recognize that our dogs may not always reciprocate this desire. Determining whether your dog loves or merely tolerates interactions with strangers is crucial. A dog that genuinely enjoys these interactions will do so effortlessly and willingly, without any prompting or need for coercion. For instance, they may be the ones to initiate contact with strangers and not just remain close to their owners in public spaces. To help illustrate this concept, I will use my two therapy dogs as examples.

I have two therapy dogs, each with a unique personality. Oreo is a younger, brilliant, and active dog. I prefer to work with her with adolescents and adults. She is highly focused on me and will only engage with individuals briefly if I am not nearby. Oreo will always ensure that I am nearby before approaching people, and once she receives the go-ahead, she will often lie down, show her belly, or request rubs.

*Aragundeu1@uagm.edu

© CAB International 2024. *Animal-assisted Interventions: Recognizing and Mitigating Potential Welfare Challenges* (ed. L.R. Kogan)
DOI: 10.1079/9781800622616.0030

In contrast, Pascuas is an older, exceptionally sweet, and mellow dog that prefers to be cute and loving rather than perform tricks. She gives love and attention to individuals, but she settles down once she finds the perfect spot for belly rubs. Pascuas is suitable for everyone but excels in working with small children and challenging conversations. Both dogs genuinely enjoy their work, evident through their willingness to walk around and connect with different people.

A lot of the work I do is with PR Animals. PR Animals has had one mission since I founded it in 2010: to educate the Puerto Rican community about compassion, kindness, and responsible guardianship. Education is the principal objective of our organization because, through it, we can provide the information that strengthens the human–animal bond and change perceptions about adopting *satos* (mutts). Our Humane Education Program is our investment in Puerto Rico's future. Empathy, compassion, kindness, pet care, and volunteer work are some values we encourage in the students who participate in our programs. We have reached over 10,000 students, teachers, police officers, and community members with programs like Educating future Educators, Remember Me Thursday™, Student Lobbying, and many more.

Typical Scenario

When coordinating any visit that includes Oreo and Pascuas, we make sure to send all the pertinent documents, including Consent, Release and Hold Harmless Agreement, and Photo Use Release Forms. When I partner with Oreo and Pascuas to enhance, exemplify, and practice knowledge about animal welfare and the human–animal bond in group settings, it is always a fantastic experience. First, participants are encouraged to connect with Oreo and Pascuas. This can be challenging in classrooms full of children, adolescents, or adults who want or ask for the dogs' attention. However, this provides an excellent opportunity to decrease people's inhibitions and increase focus and motivation. This connection also opens the possibility for interactive conversations about the need to work towards improving the lives of the homeless dogs and cats on the streets. Through storytelling, I can educate participants about the lives of Oreo

and Pascuas and the work being done to improve conditions for companion animals. I hope to foster critical thinking so that participants become future problem solvers.

When I arrive at any location, I will not let anybody engage or pet Oreo and Pascuas until I have established the rules and guidelines of interaction. This guarantees safety for all the parties involved, and I can also make sure everybody is clear about how I want them to interact with the dogs so that I can guarantee their welfare and enjoyment too.

Instructions

- First, at the beginning of any activity or intervention, I will always ask the following questions:
  - Is anybody scared of Oreo or Pascuas?
  - Would anyone feel uncomfortable if I let them walk freely around the room?
- Second, I will lay out the ground rules:
  - No running or screaming.
  - If you are not interested in engaging with the dogs, ignore them, and they will continue exploring.
  - No feeding the dogs.
  - No letting them out of the room.
  - Raise your hand if you are uncomfortable or have any concerns or questions about them.
- Third, I always include each dog's rescue story and animal-assisted therapy certification.
  - Example: Oreo and Pascuas are certified therapy dogs, and their veterinary records are current. They have been involved in our human–animal relationship work for several years, participating in workshops and events at universities, hospitals, clinics, and schools, among other places.

Monitoring during the intervention

In large group settings, I typically don't go alone and always ask someone to assist me in managing Pascuas and Oreo, checking on their well-being and interactions. This is especially important if I'm engaged in an activity that is difficult to interrupt, such as support or therapy groups. What I will do is:

- call the dogs to my side every 10 min; and
- ask the group where each dog is located (e.g. sleeping beside someone petting them) if I cannot see them immediately.

Physical location

I always try to ensure that we have a spacious room to conduct the workshop so that both the dogs and the participants can feel comfortable and have enough space to retreat if needed. When children are involved, special care is taken, and Oreo and Pascuas are kept on a leash. If we work in pairs, I ensure that my second-in-command is vigilant and supervises any interaction to identify signs of stress in the dogs.

Consent

- Once I have assessed the context, if the dogs can roam freely, I always clarify that they will engage if they want to.
- Signs include walking up to you, smelling you, or asking for affection by lying next to you, showing their belly, or putting their heads in your lap.
- If the dogs are not interested in being included in photos and selfies, I always emphasize that this is okay and not to try to coerce the dogs into doing it.

Case Example

The team (a co-facilitator, myself, Pascuas, and Oreo) arrive at a public school in an urban area of San Juan, Puerto Rico. We are shown the space where we will work with Pascuas and Oreo. After settling in the assigned classroom, we set up audio-visuals, treats, and water for the dogs. The workshop is with middle-school children, with around 30 students and three teachers. Before allowing any interaction with Pascuas and Oreo, I wait for all the children to settle down and give instructions on how to behave around the dogs:

- no screaming;
- no running; and
- no feeding the dogs.

And now the good things:

- yes, to gentle pets; and
- yes, to look.

The second thing I do is ask about the children's comfort level. They all raise their hands, saying they are comfortable, but one girl starts crying and says she feels uncomfortable around dogs. The teacher interrupts and tries to persuade the girl that nothing will happen, but we stop the activity. My questions are:

- Does she want to leave the classroom, or does she want to stay in a safe place?
- How far or close would she feel comfortable concerning her proximity to the dogs?

Once the girl answers these questions, we can reassess where she is placed in relation to the dogs to provide a safe and enjoyable environment for everyone. The best part of this experience was that she timidly asked when the activity was finished if she could touch the dogs. We made a deal that I would give them some treats so that she could gently pet them. She was very proud of herself when she left the classroom. Usually, we find that once children observe the dogs and see how well behaved they are, those who were initially afraid want to interact with them during or after the activity.

Discussion questions

1. Which stress signs do we need to watch out for in Pascuas or Oreo in this type of intervention?
2. What other things could we have done to ensure the girl's comfort level?
3. What do we do if we see children trying to give kisses to the dogs?

31 Calling Dr. Doolittle: The Clinician's Role in Monitoring Communication Between Animal and Client to Maintain Safety During Animal-assisted Psychotherapy Interventions

LINDA CHASSMAN CRADDOCK*

Animal Assisted Therapy Programs of Colorado, Arvada, Colorado, USA

Abstract

This chapter explores different challenges in determining which animal or animal species to choose in a particular animal-assisted psychotherapy (AAP) intervention. While dogs make excellent introductory animals, other prey animals can offer a greater challenge and hence growth experience for clients. How to choose an animal depends on an array of factors including the client's ability to engage safely with the animal, the treatment goal, and most importantly, the animal's well-being and willingness to engage. These things are discussed, along with how to mitigate the welfare challenges for human and animal and provide examples of ways to interrupt potentially harming behavior.

The session started outside on a sunny afternoon. I took Sean, a 32-year-old divorced man, into one of our outside therapy spaces and was immediately met by Lily. Lily was shy for a moment, and then she started her silly Lily behavior—pushing against Sean with her head and then standing up to her full 5 feet (1.5 m) to come crashing back down with another head nudge (Video 31.1).

Video 31.1

Lily's natural behavior.

https://www.cabidigital library. org/ doi/ book/ 10.1079/9781800622616. 0000

This behavior is quite normal for Lily; she is a large Nubian goat. And Lily wanted to play! Despite trying to train her to have better goat manners, Lily persists on playing with humans the same way she plays with her goat friends.

We often are asked why we have a poorly behaved therapy animal like Lily. We explain that Lily is a happy girl, and our designated "boundary training goat". As a center where we provide animal-assisted psychotherapy (AAP), our animals enjoy many roles, not all of which include creating a calm, accepting place. Our clients are often adults who have been through numerous therapies and have come to our center because other treatment modalities have not worked for them. As a clinician for over 30 years, I have become aware how limiting talking therapy can be for some clients. Here, stepping into Lily's therapy office, the client

*Lchassman@aatpc.org

is immediately challenged to either learn some new boundary-setting behaviors or get (literally) pushed around. Our goal with AAP is to provide relational experiences with animals that push the client just out of their comfort zone, while also supporting their ability to utilize their internal resources to learn. We help clients see alternative ways to think, feel, and behave that will ultimately be more successful.

Multiple welfare challenges exist when integrating any animal into work with humans. The client, the animal, and the clinician can each be negatively impacted if an intervention is not carefully considered, approached, and supervised. It is the clinician's responsibility to monitor sessions to ensure they are safe and positive for all involved.

Choosing the Animal

Having a wide range of therapy animals at our farm affords us the opportunity to carefully choose which animal will help with a particular client at a specific time in therapy and with a certain treatment goal. Due to her rambunctious behavior, Lily is not for new clients or young children. A large part of the clinician's job is to determine the relative risk to benefit ratio for integrating each of our animals into a session. The decision about which clients work with which animals is a complex but intentional process because any animal can create a safety challenge for clients, and vice versa. The animal's welfare always comes first, even if this disappoints or frustrates a client.

At our therapy farm we have horses, donkeys, alpacas, goats, chickens, dogs, cats, rabbits, rats, guinea pigs, and ferrets. The primary determination for choosing the animal for any session is whether the animal and client can interact safely. Our smallest therapy animal, our rats, are fragile and move quickly. We may not choose rats when working with clients who have a history of harming animals, or who have impulse control or motor issues. Hawk, our quarter horse, is our largest animal at over 1000 lb (454 kg) and can break a limb with a simple misstep. With large animals, it is imperative that we know in advance that the client can, and will, follow directions and rules for safe interaction.

My preference for an introductory animal is my dog, Rupert. He is an 80 lb (36 kg) Lab border collie mix. His training and socialization as a therapy dog included rough handling, loud noises, and quick movements. He can tolerate unpredictable behavior and enjoys spontaneous and rowdy playfulness. Rupert provides the attentiveness, acceptance, and positive support that clients need at the initial stages of therapy, which also makes him a great starter therapy animal.

With the exception of dogs, most of our therapy animals are prey animals that develop relationships over time as they feel safe. Learning to build relationships with these animals is both motivating and challenging for clients who need to develop empathy and understanding of others.

Determining the Intervention

Which intervention and animal we choose depends on several factors. We account for the client's interest, treatment goals, and their ability to regulate as well as the time in treatment (i.e. beginning, middle, or end). An intervention we often use with clients of all ages is animal training. All animals can be trained: for example, Rupert knows immediately what the clicker means, while the chickens are just learning to associate the click with a treat.

The most challenging, but most effective, interventions are created spontaneously as the clinician notices how an animal is responding to the client. A client, Jim, and I were talking about his current relationship problems while among the herd of horses, and he was trying to receive comfort from our horse, Cody. Cody turned, walked away, and went behind a fence. When I asked Jim what he thought had happened, he said "this felt just like what my girlfriend does, and my mother did, when I needed them. They went away and left me alone". This prompted an exploration of this pattern and how to change it; what was needed to change this pattern. Jim experimented with various ways of *being* with Cody before Cody chose to come back to his side.

The Issue of Consent

We would never ask a client to do something against their will. We must treat animals the same way. Because animals do not have the words to give verbal consent, we must know each of our animals well enough to understand how they give consent, how they remove consent, and how they just say *no*.

Each animal is different, but all have their own way of expressing the initial signs of concern/stress.

Dogs, cats, and horses use calming signals to communicate their intentions. Seeing a calming signal does not always mean "no" but it does indicate some important communication we should heed. Consent may be communicated by the animal by simply moving towards or away from the clinician and client. If an animal moves away, we honor the animal's desire to disengage and allow them to go to a neutral space. This may be outside the area, the room, in a safe kennel, or under a piece of furniture. When Rupert is stressed, he will go to the door and look at it. My job as his advocate is to open the door and let him go to a place of his choice.

Clients also need to give consent. While it may be therapeutic for the client to learn how to set boundaries with our pushy goat Lily, if they do not feel safe, the client can also decline consent. But since many clients are also non-verbal, or have difficulty expressing their feelings, the clinician needs to watch and check in around the client's stress as well.

Monitoring the Interaction for Animal and Client Safety

We evaluate clients over time to learn how they respond to directions and rules. When we find clients with uncontrollable impulsivity, angry outbursts, quick movements, or loud voices, we may opt to start with an animal representation (i.e. toy animals). Stuffed animals have helped even some adult clients practice how to safely hold, pet, and interact with various animals and give us important information about their readiness to work with a live animal.

Most of our interactions, however, involve live animals. Unless there is a separate handler, it falls to the clinician to constantly monitor the animals' behavior, and particularly watch for signs of stress. We talk about animals *whispering*, *speaking*, and then *yelling*. They whisper to us through their calming signals or non-verbal behavior. It's at that point that a clinician should stop what they are doing and decide if the animal needs a break. Waiting until the animal "speaks" is often too late; this means the animal is stressed, anxious or fearful and is only a step away from "yelling,' which is when an animal lashes out, usually in the form of

a warning bite or kick. Even a warning can cause a great deal of physical and/or emotional harm.

The clinician's job is also to protect the client from an animal's potential behavior. Lily is an example of an animal who enjoys working with clients and engaging with them in her playful way. We bring clients to Lily who are ready for the challenge she provides, but also remain close enough to coach them as needed in setting firm limits. We also get between them if necessary. Here is an example of how clients taught Lily to enjoy her goat game while also being safer with the humans (Videos 31.2 and 31.3).

Video 31.2

Lily helping clients set limits and boundaries.

https://www.cabidigital library.org/doi/book/ 10.1079/9781800622616. 0000

Video 31.3

Lily helping clients set limits and boundaries.

https://www.cabidigital library.org/doi/book/ 10.1079/9781800622616. 0000

We have learned over the years how to contain the environment in ways that increase safety. For example, we don't have dogs around when we work with the horses. We don't have young children feed the horses. When we want to work with a specific animal, we move them to a more isolated area so the other animals don't interrupt or become confused.

Interrupting the Intervention When a Potential Welfare Breach Occurs

One of the largest challenges we face is when a client wants to work with an animal, but the animal is showing signs of stress or doesn't want to engage with a client. Because we allow animals to choose when and how to interact with clients, they may behave in ways that hurt the client's feelings or frustrate them. There are other times when the human starts to engage in behavior that creates stress or discomfort for the animal.

I have had circumstances where a client's behavior quickly becomes problematic, and I have had to quickly remove the animal for its protection. This creates a difficult situation for the client. After practicing with a stuffed rat, I allowed Missy to hold Cinnamon, a 1-year-old rat. After a few moments Missy started to hold Cinnamon over her head and "fly" her around. There was not much time to think about the most therapeutic way to ask Missy to safely put Cinnamon down, so I quickly said "I'll take Cinnamon!" In order to spare Cinnamon any more stress, I had set a quick boundary with Missy that potentially created a breach in our therapeutic relationship.

Interceptions like these can be difficult, but an animal's welfare must come first. The breach in my relationship with Missy could be (and was) quickly repaired and I believe that good therapy includes the ability to repair breaches in the therapeutic relationship. I was able to help Missy to empathize with Cinnamon and understand the need for my interruption in her play. For clients who have experienced abuse, this also models appropriate care and concern. Gently helping a client to understand how an animal might feel in different circumstances is an important therapeutic goal.

Other statements I might make to regulate increasingly worrying client behavior are:

- What do you think the animal is feeling right now?
- How would you feel if you were a little animal being held very high?
- What else could you do that might make them feel safer?

Choosing when and which animals to include in treatment with each individual client is like making a new dance to a new song every session. There is no formula. But the clinician needs to: (i) know their animal(s); (ii) have good communication with their client; and (iii) find that balance between challenging the client, yet not pushing so hard they become stressed. That is the delicate dance of AAP.

Discussion Questions

1. How would you have handled the situation with Missy? What would you say if you were faced with a situation where your animal was becoming stressed by a client's behavior?
2. How does your animal demonstrate consent? How do they withdraw consent or say "no" to an invitation for interaction?
3. Do you work with an animal that uses calming signals for communication? If so, which calming signals does your animal frequently use and how can you tell when your animal is becoming more stressed?
4. Considering your primary client population and animal(s), think of three different statements you can make to clients if you need to interrupt an intervention that is becoming unsafe for them or for the animal.

32 Canine Co-therapists—Special Considerations for Engaging Within Virtual Environments and Navigating Canine Health-status Changes

Donna Clarke*

Linganore Counseling and Wellness, LLC, New Market, Maryland, USA

Abstract

With the ever-expanding telemental health component of mental health, recognizing the needs of the co-therapist, whether as a component of a virtual or *in vivo* mental health experience, remains a key factor in the journey with one's clients. This chapter seeks to examine key factors when engaging with clients in animal-assisted interventions (AAIs) both *in vivo* and within the telemental health setting.

It is important for clinicians to be ever mindful of the triad which exists within the therapeutic realm, when a co-therapist (human or animal) participates in the therapeutic journey. Within the telemental health world, several considerations pertaining to the well-being of the animal co-therapist are important to explore. The first pertains to awareness related to the therapeutic setting. As clients observe your co-therapist through your webcam, special consideration should be given to angles and lighting to provide the best opportunity for a successful visual, virtual connection between client, co-therapist, and therapist. If the co-therapist happens to be a 5.5 lb (2.5 kg) teacup poodle (as is Miss Emmie, my co-therapist) this is a much less taxing endeavor. If, however, one's co-therapist is a 40 lb (18 kg) golden retriever, or a 65 lb (29 kg) labradoodle, establishing a setting which is both comfortable and inviting for both human and canine, as well as engaging for the client, might include additional considerations related to furnishings, as well as technology. Other important aspects of care and welfare of the co-therapist whether *in vivo* or through the telemental modality include consistently available fresh, clean water and food options, as well as frequent breaks for the canine to walk, stretch, play, or rest. It is also important to be mindful of the dog's triggers and/or stressors, and what care is needed both as a frontloading strategy, as well as in the moment. This is similar to how we explore tools, strategies, and self-care with our clients. The importance of these elements cannot be overstated, as the canine co-therapist participates as an integral part of *our* journey in the world of work, not theirs. As such, our canines need to have the ability to choose whether to engage, based upon their unique needs of the day.

Beyond the basics of care for our co-therapist, is the need for clinicians to be aware of the impact of their canine co-therapist's individual journey in the therapeutic relationship. For example, absences from sessions due to scheduling changes, health issues, or necessary down time are important things to consider. When scheduling clients, it is important

*Donnac42086@gmail.com

DOI: 10.1079/9781800622616.0032

to discuss the fact that your canine co-therapist may not always be present. Talking about the needs of "Miss Emmie" and her ability to choose whether to participate has been assistive in helping clients have realistic expectations and has proven a valuable tool with clients surrounding boundaries and expectations.

Another important factor to consider when working with a canine co-therapist, whether remotely or *in vivo*, is recognizing that the dog represents different constructs to different clients. In the case of Miss Emmie, there are clients who begin each session inquiring as to her presence, status, and/or health. These discussions are often a representation and comparison of their own individual journeys. An example would be the client who typically asks if Miss Emmie is present, and had slept well the night before. I inquire with the client, based upon her perception of Miss Emmie's expression, her interpretation of Miss Emmie's restorative sleep the night before. This client shares her perceptions, which she then utilizes as a way to talk about and explore her own sleep journey, allowing her some distance to navigate her thoughts and feelings, as she shares sleep strategies with Miss Emmie.

Additionally, there are clients who attend virtual therapy sessions with their own pets. They engage in animal-assisted intervention (AAI) activities, share perceptions of positive outcomes, and connect with their pet, while observing my interactions with Miss Emmie. One client, for example, joins with her canine companion, and shares with Miss Emmie during our sessions in a way that feels more comfortable for her than talking directly to me. This client's perceptions surrounding presence and comfort, as well as the tools she utilizes for self-care, are shared among her furry family member and Miss Emmie, and provides this client with a sense of acceptance and validation.

Some clients inquire about Miss Emmie solely when she is not visually present on screen, seeking comfort in the consistency of her more passive presence. The unspoken constancy of the co-therapist is an important factor which cannot be understated. Miss Emmie is present during sessions from the vantage point of my chair—or her own individual chair. Additionally, she has a resting area and play area which is located off screen. One client, who ordinarily talks with me when Miss Emmie is sitting quietly on my chair, inquired about Miss Emmie one morning. When told that Miss Emmie was off screen in her rest area, the client sighed, visibly relieved that Miss Emmie was close and safe. The client made connections to her own loss journey, and shared perceptions surrounding the presence—and unexpected absence—of her lost loved ones.

There exists an unavoidable challenge when sharing the therapeutic journey with a canine co-therapist: the inevitable aging and death process. Clients connect with co-therapists in ways which often feel more significant—more *real*—than with others, whether family, friends, or clinicians. This can be due to perceptions of unconditional positive regard and non-judgmental presence, which only the co-therapist can truly provide. As such, clients may feel deeply impacted by the dog's health decline and/or death. It is important to be candid and proactively communicate changes whenever possible, and therapeutically appropriate. Recently Miss Emmie was scheduled for a surgical procedure. Aware of the healing process, when clinically appropriate, I journeyed with clients regarding her pending pre- and post-surgical absence, as well as convalescence. Clients expressed appreciation for the awareness, and shared their own thoughts, feelings, and wishes pertaining to her health and wellness. This experience also provided for an organic exploration of tools and strategies related to a myriad of client symptomology, from anxiety to expressions of depression, grief, and loss as a result of trauma. This discussion enabled clients to share tools they have acquired along their therapeutic journeys, including stories of healing, which in turn could be utilized to examine their individual experiences more deeply.

Clinicians share a special connection with their canine co-therapists. When navigating health changes related to their canine co-therapist, clinicians are best served to be aware of their own self-care and status, in order that they may bring best practice to their clients. To that end, it is important we are mindful of our own mental health needs when navigating the health-status shifts of our co-therapists. As our co-therapist's lifespan is sadly more finitely defined, clinician awareness of a co-therapist's potential retirement and/or aging process can be valuable, as well as a component of best practice when negotiating potential confounds and triggers related to a client's history of loss and trauma. To be sure, these are conversations which are potentially triggering for the clinician, as well as the client. Self-awareness as well as utilization of both supervision and support systems can be assistive in maintaining presence and attunement for your clients.

The unique relationship of the therapist, canine co-therapist, and client provides a special opportunity to delicately explore client thoughts, feelings, and perceptions surrounding aspects of their individual journeys. In that regard, the perception of the client pertaining to health shifts of the dog may involve exploration of deeply complex thoughts and feelings. Navigating loss is a unique journey which, as Kessler (2021) so eloquently states, is as "individual as a fingerprint". Clinician awareness that the loss of the canine co-therapist can provoke complicated feelings and thoughts for the client is critical. It is important for the clinician to process their own thoughts, feelings, and grief pertaining to health shifts and/or loss related to the canine co-therapist, in order to maintain presence and attunement with the client, as they examine the client's individual perceptions. This cannot be overly emphasized. Special consideration and care related to the clinician's individual grief journey is an important factor, especially when addressing loss and grief with clients. Being mindful of the client's grief history and process, and endeavoring to remain present in the client's experience can be further codified by clinician self-care, self-awareness, and of course processing of their own individual grief, and grief/loss journeys. As a colleague of mine so eloquently states, "therapists are people too". Taking time to check-in and process one's own grief and loss is an integral and necessary part of being present for your client's journey through their processing of potential grief and loss, and the canine co-therapist.

Discussion Questions

1. In what ways can a therapist assist a client to navigate health decline/shifts of the co-therapist? What are potential triggers for either the client or the clinician?
2. In what ways can the therapist maintain presence and attunement with the client when navigating health-status shifts and/or loss of the co-therapist? What tools/strategies might one use?

Reference

Kessler, D. (2021) *Unattended Grief: Interventions to Facilitate Healthy Grieving*. Digital Seminar (Online). The Grief Summit: Grief Counseling and Treatment in a Pandemic of Loss, April 29–April 30, PESI, Eau Claire, Wisconsin.

33 Animal Welfare with AAI in Prisons/Jails

Yvonne Eaton-Stull*

Slippery Rock University, Slippery Rock, Pennsylvania, USA

Abstract

For some people, visiting a locked facility like a jail or prison causes concern and anxiety. Yet, volunteers and workers who choose to engage in this line of work realize the potential risks and deem them acceptable in relation to the potential benefits. Our therapy dogs, however, do not have these same choices. Therefore, it is up to us, as the professionals, to assure that any and all risks and concerns be adequately addressed to make sure our animal's physical and mental well-being is protected at all times. Over the past 8 years, I have engaged in animal-assisted social work interventions in various jails, prisons, and juvenile facilities. In this chapter I share various animal welfare challenges, along with strategies I have utilized to manage and mitigate such risks, specifically related to therapy dogs.

Selection of Dogs and Handlers

Many people have heard the saying that stress and emotions of handlers can go right down the leash to affect the dog. Therefore, it is essential for canine handlers to be calm and comfortable in a locked facility. It is important to know what is being asked of both the handler and the canine, including length of time, roles and duties, clearances needed, security processes, and behavioral expectations. When I was developing a team of handlers to offer services in locked facilities, I was fortunate to know many great therapy dog handlers. I explained what I was looking for, answered questions, and obtained their commitment. For those who are starting a program from scratch, I would strongly suggest meeting both handler and dog to assure they have the personality and temperament for what you are looking for. Ideally, meeting them in the secure facility would provide an opportunity to observe obvious stress signs or concerns prior to implementing the animal-assisted intervention (AAI). For the handler, I would likely pose such questions as:

- Have you ever been in a jail/prison?
- What concerns do you have about being locked inside a facility?
- What are *your* stress signs?
- How do you know when your dog is stressed?
- What do you do to manage your own/your dog's stress?

For the therapy dog, it is very important that they are extremely resilient and adaptable to environmental stressors and changes as well as various people. In my case, I often try to utilize dogs who are not only therapy dogs but also part of HOPE Animal-Assisted Crisis Response (AACR) teams. I do this for a variety of reasons. The HOPE AACR teams have to pass an extensive screening to determine aptitude for responding to stressful situations; this evaluation is much longer and more intense than typical therapy dog tests. The tests provide a simulated roleplay with a great deal of environmental noises and stimuli. Additionally, the HOPE AACR teams' intensive 3-day certification provides training in both human and canine stress management. Finally, these teams are required to

*yvonne.eaton-stull@sru.edu

© CAB International 2024. *Animal-assisted Interventions: Recognizing and Mitigating Potential Welfare Challenges* (ed. L.R. Kogan)
DOI: 10.1079/9781800622616.0033

complete annual continuing education training which enhances their knowledge and skill in both canine behavior/handling and human needs/crisis intervention.

Environmental Stressors

There are numerous, unusual stressors in jails/prisons which both handlers and dogs will encounter. Walking through metal detectors present a challenge when the handler must clear the device before calling the dog through. In some cases, handheld metal detectors are also used which can be scary for a dog who is unfamiliar with this object. Practice run throughs can be valuable in assuring smooth, efficient processes. Very heavy, loud clanging sliding doors are another experience which present a significant risk to a dog's tail if they don't clear the doors in time. Again, practice exposures will help both handlers and dogs to know what to expect. Many secure facilities also have escape whistles or alarms on a regular basis which may startle or induce fear in a dog. Ensuring handlers have high-value treats for these occurrences can help them create a positive association with these sounds for their dog.

Men and women in uniform, weapons, and varied floor surfaces or stairs may be unfamiliar to dogs. Early exposure to these diverse experiences can help a dog gain confidence and flexibility when responding to different environments. These secure environments also have procedures to verify and count those in custody; these "count times" may result in lock downs for periods of time when the institution is attempting to verify inconsistencies. Handlers should be made aware of this potential situation. These lock-down periods require patience and flexibility for those involved. Asking potential handlers how they would handle these types of situations can be helpful in determining their suitability for work inside locked facilities.

One other environmental stressor often present in cold climates is snow and ice. Salt utilized on these surfaces is often not pet safe: it can be caustic and burn a dog's feet. Making sure the handler has a towel and supplies to wipe their dog's feet is essential in this case.

Logistics

Determining where AAI should be held in a facility is an important logistical issue to assure handlers and dogs are comfortable and safe. The size of a room is something to consider so that all involved do not feel cramped or distressed. The rooms that are most comfortable typically are large rooms with two exits with windowed doors for security officers to periodically observe and monitor any safety issues. It is important to have enough space for individuals to be able to sit on the floor to interact with the dogs if they desire. A circle of chairs on the perimeter of the room works much better than a room with a conference table in the center.

Some facilities have metal steps or open steps (without backs); these can be problematic for some dogs to navigate. A room on a ground floor is a great way to avoid these challenges. A few facilities I have worked in also provide personal alarms that are secured on your body. One time, however, my dog Chevy dislodged the alarm, causing a reaction by the incarcerated men to put their hands in the air and back up against a wall. Knowing what to do in the event of a crisis is essential for anyone working in these facilities.

I have found between eight and ten (no more than 12) attendees to be a good number for a group session with two dogs and their handlers present. Making sure that the dogs have met before the first day is essential as you want to have dogs who get along but prefer interaction with people versus each other. It is also essential to ask the facility what times must be avoided, for example: mealtimes, count times, and shift changes should be avoided if possible. It is also helpful to have extra time before the start of your group session to allow ample time for participants to clear security checkpoints and get to the AAI location. For example, although the actual group session may be from 10 a.m. to 11 a.m., 9:45 a.m. is put on the appointment schedule for participants.

It is also helpful to have about four approved therapy dog teams to utilize. Although I only use two at any given time, it is helpful to have backups in the case of cancellations or if it is necessary to replace one due to showing too much stress. Constant monitoring of the dogs for obvious stress signs is essential. Excessive panting, pulling away, shaking, and whining can be indicative of distress. Taking immediate action to address stress in the therapy dogs can include taking them out for a break, giving them a drink/treat, or ending the visit early for that team.

It is also important to take the time to develop explicit exclusionary criteria for those who should not be permitted to attend any AAI sessions. I always exclude any individuals with a known history of cruelty to animals. Also, I exclude anyone with a recent history (in the last 6 months) of violence toward others. It is essential to develop great relationships with the staff in these facilities; they know the clients well and can be helpful partners in screening participants in advance of implementation.

As a social worker, it is my job to assure the safety of my clients and when providing AAIs, my concerns extend to the therapy dogs and handlers with whom I work. Taking preventative actions to protect the physical and mental well-being of *all* participants is essential to ensure freedom from fear, distress, discomfort, pain, and injury while enhancing the care and treatment provided.

Case Example I

Going inside a prison or jail often requires pre-approval for anything being brought inside the facility. There are many excluded items as well, including but not limited to cellphones, gum, lighters, smart watches, liquids, and medication. Furthermore, everything is searched, which can delay the process for getting inside to begin a program.

Discussion questions

1. What are things that might be needed when bringing a therapy dog into a jail/prison?
2. What things would you need to remove or not provide to those who are incarcerated when implementing AAI?

Case Example II

Developing policies and criteria for an AAI is essential for the safe implementation and success of a program. Just because an agency requests a particular group or intervention doesn't mean it is a good idea. I have been asked to provide an animal-assisted anger management group, but due to fear of impulsivity and dangers to my dog, I have declined.

Discussion questions

1. If you were going to provide an animal-assisted anger management group: (a) What would you have for your inclusion criteria? (b) What size of group would you recommend? (c) Are there any behaviors and/or diagnoses you would exclude?
2. What considerations would you have for the therapy dog(s)?

34 The InterProfessional Animal-assisted Wellness (IPAW) Collaborative

LAURA POLESHUCK* AND MISSY REED

Nazareth University, Rochester, New York, USA

Abstract
This chapter explores the strategies used to ensure animal and human welfare in a campus-integrated therapy dog program at a small liberal arts and professional university with 2550 undergraduate and graduate students and two therapy dog–faculty-member handler teams.

Guiding Eyes for the Blind Proposal, Fall Semester 2019

Like many college/university faculty and staff members, I, Laura, became aware of the high rates of anxiety, depression, and stress in students during my first 6 years of teaching at the undergraduate and graduate levels. By reviewing the literature and pulling from prior experience implementing animal-assisted activities and therapy, I knew that interaction with dogs can improve college-student mood, energy, and well-being, and decrease anxiety, increasing students' ability to participate in academic and social aspects of the college experience. I wanted to bring some of those benefits to our campus in a judicious manner, simultaneously respecting the University's values of service and inclusion. I decided to propose that I become a puppy raiser for Guiding Eyes for the Blind (GEB). Thus began the path that resulted in a campus-integrated therapy dog program (Fig. 34.1).

GEB breeds their own dogs for traits that will be necessary in their future work as service dogs, including a calm and friendly demeanor and excellent learning ability. Thus I felt that a partnership between the University community and GEB would provide an excellent physical and social environment for a guide dog in training, expose students, staff, and faculty to a friendly puppy and an outstanding program, and potentially help meet the needs of someone who is blind. In the summer of 2020, GEB puppy Orion began visiting campus with me to become familiar with the environment (Fig. 34.2).

From the outset, I implemented several strategies to ensure the welfare of both Orion and the many students, faculty, and staff.

- *Preparation*: Orion did not come to campus until she was fully vaccinated and had passed the behavioral tests required to earn her GEB puppy in training vest. She wore the vest at all times to indicate that she was not a pet and belonged in indoor spaces.
- *Education*:
  o An article about Orion and GEB was placed in the school's e-newsletter; it invited people to reach out with questions/concerns.
  o Students, faculty, and staff who chose to engage with Orion were educated on proper interactions.

*Corresponding author: Lpolesh3@naz.edu

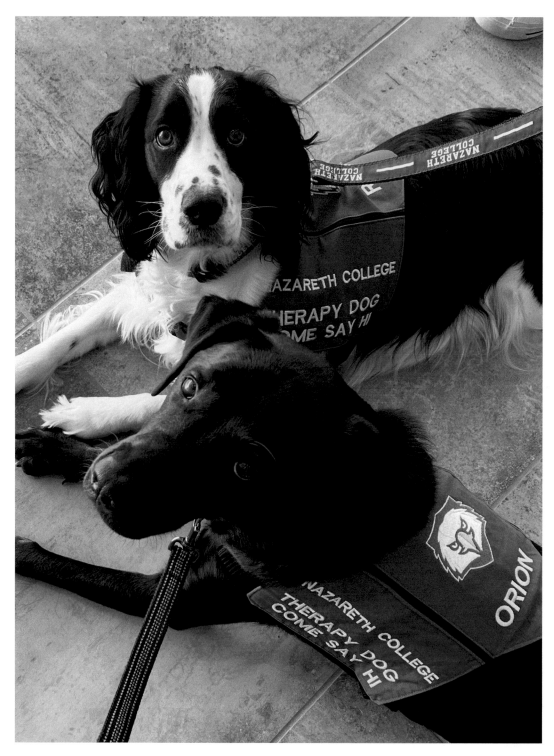

Fig. 34.1. Therapy dogs Orion and Rosie at Nazareth College (now Nazareth University).

L. Poleshuck and M. Reed

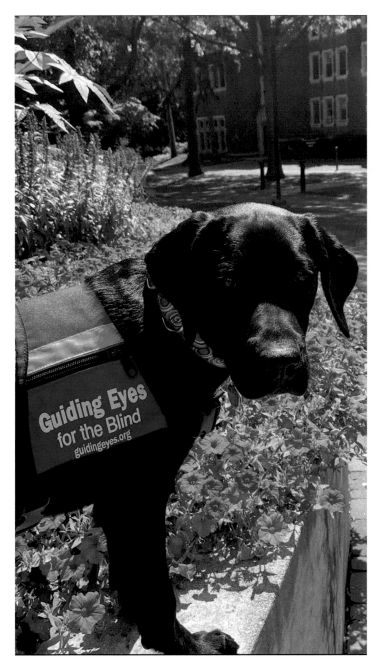

Fig. 34.2. Orion visiting campus.

○ Students who helped to walk Orion as part of a GEB-approved research study were given a 2-hour long orientation which included practice with handling Orion and working on her training skills.

● *Daily schedule*: On a daily basis, Orion was provided with multiple walks, opportunities to play, and time to rest away from others. From a young age she had exposure to wheelchairs/ walkers, various human and mechanical noises, and people of all ages and abilities/disabilities due to my office's vicinity to our on-campus occupational, physical, speech, and creative arts therapy clinics.

I disseminated a "Dog on Campus" survey in November 2020 to students and full-time staff and faculty members. Of the 746 participants, 90% said that they did not have any concerns about a dog being on campus. Concerns that were noted by the other 10% primarily included allergies, cleanliness, poor behavior, and concerns for people who fear dogs. All of these factors are important to consider when incorporating a dog into a campus community, and efforts to ameliorate such effects were already in place and continue. For example: (i) Orion's hair and teeth are brushed daily; (ii) all waste is removed promptly and put into a dumpster, not a garbage can; (iii) students are informed before each semester begins that I am planning on bringing Orion to class, and are invited to voice any concerns; and (iv) Orion remains on leash in class unless all students vote (anonymously) for me to allow her to move about the classroom. Despite the concerns noted, over 99% of the survey respondents recognized benefits to having a dog on campus. Another survey conducted in November 2022 demonstrated that the vast majority of students (97%) had no concerns about the dogs being on campus, suggesting that our strategies have been successful.

Orion Proposal, Fall Semester 2020

At 9 months old, Orion's skills and manners were blossoming, and she had participated in a research project with first-year students having positive results related to their retention and academic success. However, she had repeated ear infections and was released from the GEB program for medical issues. I agreed to adopt Orion, and in a second evidence-based proposal I suggested that Orion become a therapy dog who could: (i) continue her meaningful daily interactions with students in and out of the classroom; (ii) continue to participate in research on animal-assisted interventions; and (iii) engage with community participants in on-campus therapeutic and educational clinics and programs. Orion and I became a Pet Partners-registered therapy dog–handler team in July 2021. In 2022, the Association of Animal-Assisted Intervention Professionals (AAAIP) grew out of Pet Partners; it offers education, certification,

networking, and insurance, all of which are essential to ensure welfare and ethical practices. I earned the accompanying Animal-Assisted Intervention Specialist Certification (C-AAIS) in 2022 and have been a member of AAAIP since its inception.

Rosie Proposal, Summer 2021

Due to the growing number of potential activities and projects for Orion on campus, one dog was no longer sufficient to meet the demand while maintaining animal welfare. I, Missy, a full-time faculty member of 5 years, had been training my puppy Rosie for the American Kennel Club® S.T.A.R. Puppy certification, which entails many of the skills needed to become a registered therapy dog. I had similar concerns to those voiced by Laura about the state of student mental health on campus, and recognized that this was exacerbated by coronavirus disease 2019 (COVID-19). Laura and I proposed that Rosie start in the summer of 2021 to acclimate her to the campus environment. In a third evidence-based proposal we noted that an additional faculty member and dog would allow us to ensure that Orion maintains a balance of participation in campus activities with play and rest and may open additional opportunities for student engagement and research. That summer Rosie and Orion spent many hours together expending their puppy energy and enthusiasm and learning to behave calmly in one another's presence. Allowing them to have frequent play sessions was essential to their success in being on campus in the same building for the start of the fall semester (Fig. 34.3).

The IPAW Collaborative Is Formed, Fall and Spring Semesters 2021–2022

Now that we were both registered therapy dog–handler teams and Rosie and Orion could coexist calmly, it was time to formalize our program. We named our unique campus-integrated therapy dog program the *InterProfessional Animal-assisted Wellness (IPAW) Collaborative* to emphasize a team approach to well-being for animals and humans. Orion and Rosie began wearing vests indicating that they are therapy dogs with the University's name, colors, and mascot. Originally the vests read "please pet me"; however, in an effort to promote the importance of consent from the dogs before being touched, we changed the wording to "come say hi" (Fig. 34.1).

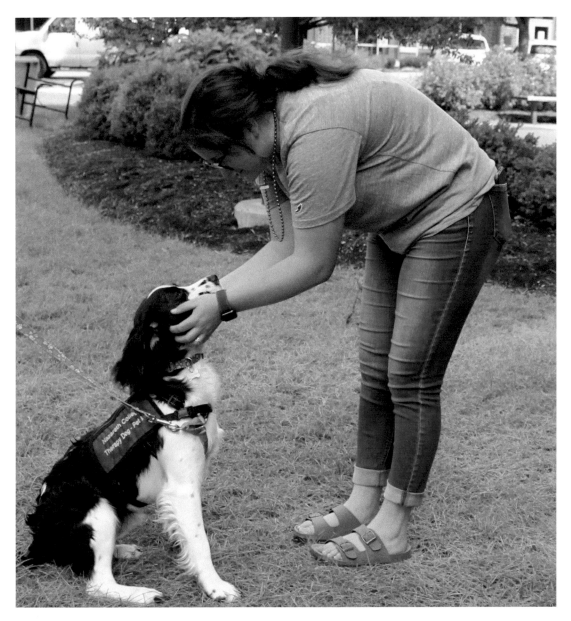

Fig. 34.3. Rosie on campus.

Each dog has comfortable spaces both inside and outside of their respective faculty member's office, and are clipped to a long line which allows them to choose between greeting students, faculty, staff, and clients just outside of the offices (Fig. 34.4) or resting inside the offices where they will not be disturbed (Fig. 34.5). The lines are short enough, however, that people can walk down the hall without having to interact with a dog, making interaction optional for both the dogs and the people. Both of our desks are situated to allow for all interactions to be supervised.

An additional space was created during this time in the library, at our request. This IPAW Pad is a dog-friendly space large enough for the dogs to chase and wrestle during our climate's many

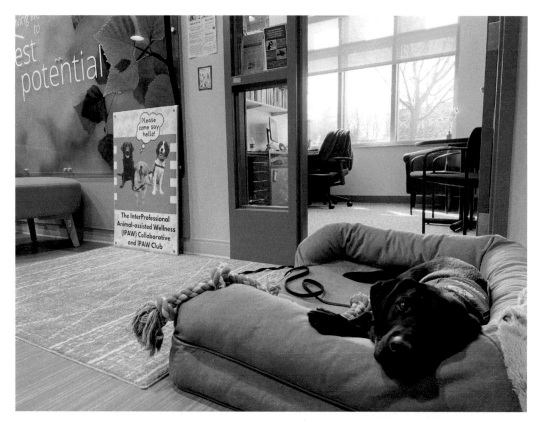

Fig. 34.4. Orion laying outside the office.

cold, hot, and rainy days. On the floor are several beanbag chairs, and there are dog toys, water, and training treats available.

The majority of student–therapy dog interactions take place in the hallway alcoves just outside of our offices, in the IPAW Pad, and on walks across campus; these spaces are part of Orion and Rosie's daily routines, and thus allow for low-stress and high-reward interactions. The dogs also attend campus events at various locations; whenever possible they are exposed to the physical space ahead of time in order to acclimate, and we remove them when they demonstrate signs of stress or fatigue or if the temperature, noise, or density of people may be counterproductive to their well-being. If a student, staff, or faculty member interacts with one of the dogs in a manner that could be distressing, we educate and advocate; however, this is an extremely rare occurrence.

Once they became registered therapy dogs, Orion and Rosie began to participate in student-run activities with clients from the community in our on-campus clinics. In order to ensure both human and animal welfare, all sessions utilize the diamond method (see Chapter 23, this volume), meaning that we function as dog handlers and not as professors or therapists during the activities. The steps detailed in Fig. 34.6 are taken before a session occurs.

During therapy sessions (e.g. Fig. 34.7) we work to ensure the welfare of the dogs, clients, student therapists, family members, and/or instructors. Because clients are selected carefully and treatment plans are discussed in advance we can focus solely on being handlers during interventions. Given this preparation, intervention for human behavior that may put the dogs' welfare at risk is needed only rarely and typically takes the form of gentle suggestions, such as where to pet the dog.

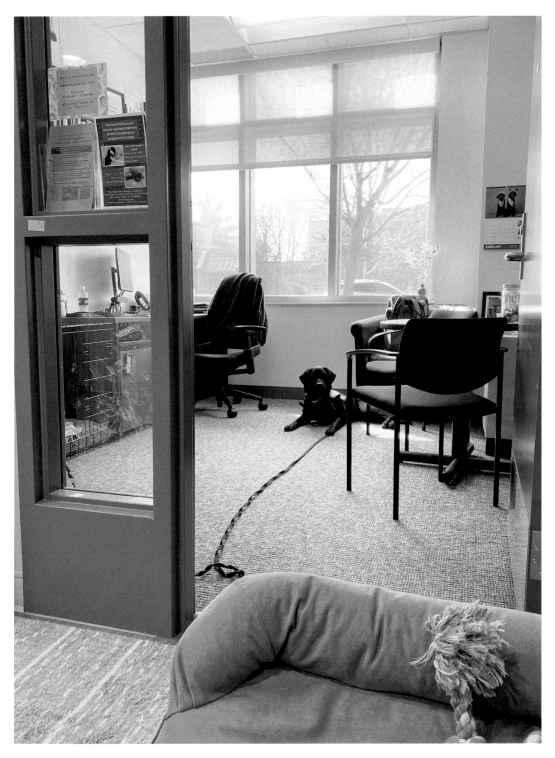

Fig. 34.5. Orion laying inside the office.

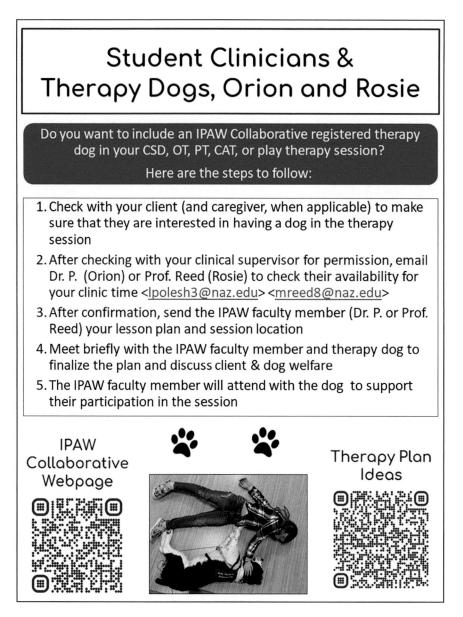

Student Clinicians & Therapy Dogs, Orion and Rosie

Do you want to include an IPAW Collaborative registered therapy dog in your CSD, OT, PT, CAT, or play therapy session?
Here are the steps to follow:

1. Check with your client (and caregiver, when applicable) to make sure that they are interested in having a dog in the therapy session
2. After checking with your clinical supervisor for permission, email Dr. P. (Orion) or Prof. Reed (Rosie) to check their availability for your clinic time <lpolesh3@naz.edu> <mreed8@naz.edu>
3. After confirmation, send the IPAW faculty member (Dr. P. or Prof. Reed) your lesson plan and session location
4. Meet briefly with the IPAW faculty member and therapy dog to finalize the plan and discuss client & dog welfare
5. The IPAW faculty member will attend with the dog to support their participation in the session

IPAW Collaborative Webpage

Therapy Plan Ideas

Fig. 34.6. Steps taken before a session occurs. CAT, creative arts therapy; CSD, communication sciences and disorders; IPAW, InterProfessional Animal-assisted Wellness; OT, occupational therapy; PT, physical therapy.

Survey, Fall Semester 2022

In November 2022 we sent out another "Dog on Campus" survey to students. We asked for students' level of agreement with the following, "The therapy dogs are treated well by their faculty handlers" and "The therapy dogs are treated well by students, staff, and faculty". A full 95.7% of respondents agreed or strongly agreed with both of these statements. We also asked students to "Please share your thoughts on Nazareth having campus-integrated therapy dogs as opposed to animal visitation programs", to which several students answered with welfare-related responses. For example:

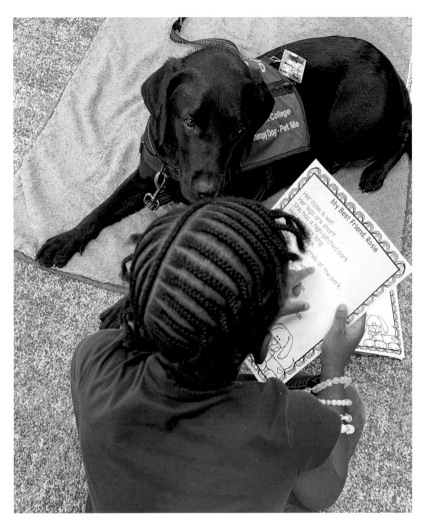

Fig. 34.7. A child reading to Orion.

I think having the integrated therapy dogs enhances the experiences because students and faculty can form more of a relationship with them by seeing the same dogs and handlers frequently. Also, it is probably nice for the dogs to spend most of their time on campus so they can be comfortable there … without always adjusting to different settings.

(Student 1)

I love the impact they make to Naz's community culture day to day and they truly have a positive impact on so many students' lives throughout the day, without adding any extra time or transportation burden onto the students or the animals.

(Student 2)

Creating the IPAW Collaborative with intentionality has allowed us to develop programs that respect the needs and priorities of our dogs while bringing joy and meaning to students, faculty, staff, and clients on campus.

Case Example

Laura and Missy have arranged their offices so the dogs may choose to be in the hallway if they wish to interact with students, faculty, staff, and community members. Each dog also has access to their crate, toys, and water within their offices. Clear signage requests that people respect the dogs' boundaries, informing them that occasionally the dogs may need a break from interacting with others, and that when the dogs are in their crates to please leave them alone.

A student enters the hallway and, not seeing Orion, calls her name. Orion remains in her office, in her crate, with the crate door open. The office door is open, with the faculty member/handler sitting at her desk. The student walks in, sits in front of the crate, and reaches in to pet Orion.

Discussion questions

1. How should the faculty member/handler respond?
2. How could this scenario be prevented in the future?

35 Safeguarding the Welfare of Therapy Dogs in Clinical Mental Health Practice

Elizabeth Ruegg*

Saint Leo University, St. Leo, Florida, USA

Abstract

This chapter explores strategies designed to safeguard the welfare of registered therapy dogs who join their guardian-handler in her animal-assisted psychotherapy practice. Show-bred female golden retrievers are described as ideal therapy dogs due to their sociability, biddability, and stability of temperament. Early social and environmental exposure practices are delineated to develop puppies for working life, along with ethical behavior training to prepare them for advanced obedience and therapy dog testing. Strategies to obtain consent from the dog for participation in therapy activities are detailed, and the identification of canine body language to communicate excitement, comfort, or stress is explained. Thoughtful decisions around the use of office space and daily scheduling are presented as means of maintaining sensitivity to working dogs' needs and welfare.

Safeguarding the Welfare of Therapy Dogs in Clinical Mental Health Practice

I have been a licensed mental health provider for over 35 years and have been incredibly fortunate in my career to merge my love for dogs and my passion for psychotherapy. After lots of study, training, and practice, I earned two credentials in animal-assisted interventions and am proud to call myself an animal-assisted psychotherapist.

Including a therapy dog in clinical practice may sound like lots of fun, but it should not be undertaken lightly. Long-term planning and significant resource investments are needed to build and maintain an effective, ethical, and liability-conscious animal-assisted psychotherapy (AAP) practice. When done well, AAP supports animal welfare and can benefit clients who struggle to succeed in traditional therapy. When done poorly, however, it may cause physical or emotional harm and increase the provider's exposure to malpractice litigation.

Because I am an experienced AAP provider, I've been asked for advice by colleagues who experienced adverse outcomes after inviting their pets to work. In one case, the dog pawed an elderly client on blood thinners, causing a skin tear that evolved into a significant wound. In another, the dog growled and barked at clients while ensconced on his guardian-handler's lap, which led clients to complain that they felt unsafe. We can infer from the dog's behavior that he felt unsafe, too.

Preparation is essential when including therapy dogs in clinical work. Virtually everything matters: (i) puppy selection and training; (ii) office space; and (iii) knowledge of canine body language, and more. Although it is a costly and time-consuming process, the benefits are immeasurable. My dogs enhance what I do as the therapist, and in some situations, they do what I cannot, such as providing physical comfort to distressed clients. Properly trained dogs who pair up with their appropriately credentialed guardian-handlers can form immensely successful

*Elizabeth.ruegg@saintleo.edu

© CAB International 2024. *Animal-assisted Interventions: Recognizing and Mitigating Potential Welfare Challenges* (ed. L.R. Kogan)
DOI: 10.1079/9781800622616.0035

psychotherapy teams to help clients achieve their treatment goals.

Ideal Dogs

Therapy dogs may be any breed, but they must have a rare combination of skills and temperament to thrive in a clinical setting. They must be biddable, accept human leadership, and prioritize human companionship. They should be responsive but not reactive, offering reliable behavior even in the presence of agitated or distressed people. Finally, they should enjoy interacting with others in addition to their guardian-handlers. Thoughtful puppy selection and training are essential to the animal's welfare because they increase the chances that each puppy will thrive in their life and career.

Labradors and golden retrievers are particularly well suited for therapy work. Goldens from show lines are my ideal choice because their light golden coats, feathered tails, and broad smiles have nearly universal appeal. They're sociable, calm, eager to learn, and quick to train. I prefer females because they are less distractable than males and do not engage in problematic behavior such as mounting or urine marking. Unlike field-bred goldens, with their high energy and prey drive, show-bred goldens enjoy physical activity yet are equally happy spending quiet hours being brushed or cuddled.

I select puppies thoughtfully. My last two generations, which include four dogs over a 13-year timespan, have come from an elite, show-line breeding program that places golden retriever pups in programs and homes where they are trained as service, show, or therapy dogs. Their genetic heritage of stable temperament, biddability, and sociability increases the likelihood that they will mature into confident, successful companions and co-workers.

I introduce my new pups to the world from their earliest weeks through novel play experiences. They romp on grass, gravel, tile, slippery marble, swaying docks, sand, asphalt, and carpet. They climb puppy-sized slides, race through fabric tunnels, hop over low hoops, and splash in shallow pools. They meet 100 friendly people in their first 100 days (yes, I count them!). These activities provide the pups with dose-controlled, confidence-enhancing, positive experiences to help them avoid phobic responses and behavioral problems later in life.

Once the pups are 4 months old, we start puppy kindergarten. Group lessons are essential for them to encounter and make friends with other people and dogs. We remain in obedience school through Canine Good Citizen training, then proceed to therapy dog formation classes until we pass the therapy dog certification test. Afterward, we visit libraries, hospitals, and schools so the pups can interact with others and carry themselves confidently in various settings. We work, train, and play together daily until they are 18 months old, by which time they are usually ready to begin work at my office.

Ideal Clients

AAP holds great promise as an adjunctive mental health intervention, but it isn't appropriate for everyone. For example, I don't consider it for clients who are aggressive, fearful of, or allergic to dogs. I also avoid it for clients with conduct disorder, antisocial personality disorder, or intermittent explosive disorder because people with these diagnoses struggle with impulse control and might act out in endangering ways.

Cultural considerations are also important. Dog ownership is most prevalent among higher-income white people in the USA (Kiefer *et al.*, 2013). So, dogs as therapy adjuncts may be more familiar and acceptable among that demographic group. By contrast, those from minoritized black, brown, and Indigenous populations have long been harassed by police dogs weaponized through attack training (Schiavone, 2019). Therefore, they may be less comfortable with a dog's participation in therapy. Similarly, people from some Asian or Middle Eastern cultures may view dogs as unclean or a food resource (Podberscek, 2009), making them inappropriate as therapy adjuncts for people with those customs and beliefs.

Obtaining Consent

Healthcare providers in the USA are legally required to obtain patients' informed consent for treatment, disclosing the intervention's risks, benefits, side effects, and alternatives. Dogs cannot verbally agree to participate in therapy activities, of course. Still, I solicit their consent to participate by presenting each dog with her working gear, which includes a site-specific collar and bandana. Each gear set is used for a single location, so the dog can scent it to learn if we are going to the library, the hospital, or the practice. She consents with her body language by wagging her tail high and fast, nosing the gear, and trotting ahead of me toward the car. Her body language tells me she declines to participate when she shows disinterest or avoidance by looking or walking away, dropping her head, or lowering her tail.

My dogs rarely decline to work. However, I recall an incident from several years ago in which Lucy, one of my most gifted therapy dogs, signaled an unwillingness to go to the office with me one morning by walking away from her presented gear. She seemed fine, and she usually loved going to the office, so I was puzzled by her behavior. However, I respected her decision and left her behind. By noon, I received a text from home reporting that Lucy had had loose stools all morning. She had *looked* fine that morning, but she clearly hadn't *felt* fine. This was an excellent reminder to me of the importance of asking for consent before each and every therapeutic encounter.

Office Space and Daily Schedule

My practice is in a former bank with a large, grassy sideyard and an expansive outdoor training area. A town park with walking trails, benches, and other amenities is across the street. The setting is perfect for AAP: we use the indoor and outdoor property, and the park across the street to engage in therapeutic activities.

I typically see five clients a day, 3 days a week. The first three sessions are followed by a 1-hour break, then we have the final two sessions before leaving the office. The dogs' rest, play, and relief breaks are built into the daily schedule. They work 1 hour at a time—no back-to-back scheduling is permitted—for a maximum of three sessions daily. When they're not working, they relax in their break room, the former tellers' station. This ample, private space is stocked with fresh water, toys, and sleeping mats to ensure their comfort.

Monitoring Communication

Dogs use body language as a non-verbal form of communication. They indicate their emotions through vocalizations, mouth shape, facial expression, body posture, and positioning of the ears and tail. As their guardian-handler, I am responsible for reading my dogs' body language to monitor their welfare and ensure they feel safe and relaxed. When happy, they wave their tails widely above their bodies, allow their tongues to loll out of their open mouths, or lean into me with their head, shoulders, or flank. When anxious or stressed, they may sniff, lick themselves compulsively, or avoid eye contact with others while maintaining a persistent help-seeking gaze (Cavalli *et al.*, 2019) with me.

When I notice this communication in session, I respond by altering the situation. For example, I might engage the dog in a quick game of catch so she can discharge her physical tension or rub her body briskly while explaining her body language to the client. Relating my recognition of the dog's stress to the client's life experience is often valuable. I might ask the client when they commonly experience stress and who is most likely to notice. I ask them to forecast how the dog probably feels when her anxiety is recognized and she is helped to become calm. In this way, the dog's experience can be a useful mirror for the client and is an effective means by which the client can gain insight into their own emotional and social experiences. Finally, if the dog remains flustered or unsettled, I don't hesitate to excuse her from the session to relax in her break room. In every situation, I'm careful to balance the needs and welfare of the client and the dog, ensuring that I fulfill my responsibility to both.

Discussion Questions

1. This chapter's introductory section described two scenarios in which therapists brought their pets to work with unfortunate results. What should those therapists have done differently to protect their dog's and clients' welfare?
2. In this chapter's "Ideal Dogs" section, the author describes her systematic process for exposing puppies to novel stimuli. How does this enhance the dogs' confidence and stability later in life?
3. In this chapter's "Office Space" section, the author describes a professional setting and schedule arranged for the comfort and welfare of her dogs. How can providers safeguard their animal's comfort and welfare if they work in a less ideal situation, such as a shared office, a smaller space, or limited access to the outdoors?

References

Cavalli, C., Carballo, F., Dzik, M.V. and Bentosela, M. (2019) Gazing as a help requesting behavior: a comparison of dogs participating in animal-assisted interventions and pet dogs. *Animal Cognition* 23(1), 141–147. DOI: 10.1007/s10071-019-01324-8.

Kiefer, V., Grogan, K.B., Chatfield, J., Glaesemann, J., Hill, W. *et al.* (2013) Cultural competence in veterinary practice. *Journal of the American Veterinary Medical Association* 243(3), 326–328. DOI: 10.2460/javma.243.3.326.

Podberscek, A.L. (2009) Good to pet and eat: the keeping and consuming of dogs and cats in South Korea. *Journal of Social Issues* 65(3), 615–632. DOI: 10.1111/j.1540-4560.2009.01616.x.

Schiavone, A.L. (2019) K-9 catch-22: the impossible dilemma of using police dogs in apprehension of suspects. *University of Pittsburgh Law Review* 80(3). DOI: 10.5195/lawreview.2019.630.

E. Ruegg

36 The Power of Non-verbal Communication

SHIRA SMILOVICI*

Prepa ibero and Clínica de Psicoterapia Asistida por Animales (CLIPA) AAT, Lerma, Mexico

Abstract

Animal-assisted psychoanalytic psychotherapy allows animals to work as co-therapists to bring to light unconscious patient processes. The spontaneous and loving behaviors of dogs add a physical element to the emotional element provided by the therapist, creating a deep bond between the patient, the therapist, and the dog. In this therapeutic process, all of the beings involved play an important part, therefore everyone's safety must be carefully protected.

A therapeutic dog is one that has the ability to provide an ambiance of complete acceptance, a non-judgmental social interaction: inducing calm, giving security, and offering confidence during difficult times. Therapeutic dogs often express acceptance, happiness, and joy which can facilitate spontaneous behaviors and feelings from patients who may not have had the same response from others during their developmental process. The non-verbal connection between humans and animals offers, to many patients, the opportunity to safely bond to another living being. The unconditional love that is expressed by therapeutic dogs allows the patients to feel welcome within the therapeutic space.

A therapy dog should be trained and able to model good behavior and create rapport with patients. They should help provide a warm, accepting setting yet also model appropriate boundaries. It is helpful if therapy dogs know some basic commands (i.e. sit, stay, come, and lay down). It is even better if they know how to greet, offer their paw to shake a human's hand, and perform other behaviors that can facilitate and promote social connections with patients. One of the most important factors within animal-assisted psychoanalytic psychotherapy is the relationship between the therapy dog and the

therapist. This relationship has to be so close that they can both predict what the other one is going to do: promoting safety for everyone who is a part of the therapeutic setting. This type of bond and communication between dog and therapist allows the dog to act freely, be spontaneous, and connect with patients.

Before beginning animal-assisted psychoanalytic psychotherapy, it is important to notify the patient about the presence of the dog. Inform them what the dog will be doing. For example, you might tell them that the dog will be freely walking around, and approaching them, or laying with/by them if they choose. Tell patients that they are allowed (and even encouraged) to talk to, play with, and pet the dog, but they must be aware that if the dog does not want to engage, they need to allow the dog its own space. Help them identify signs that might indicate the dog needs some space. The dog should be introduced, by name, as a co-therapist, and after the introduction, the dog should be allowed to behave as freely as possible.

Often, patients project onto both the dog and the therapist their feelings and thoughts. When providing animal-assisted psychoanalytic psychotherapy, one of the many goals is for the therapist, the

---

*sc.shira@gmail.com

© CAB International 2024. *Animal-assisted Interventions: Recognizing and Mitigating Potential Welfare Challenges* (ed. L.R. Kogan)
DOI: 10.1079/9781800622616.0036

animal, and the patient to form a bond that allows transference to take place. This allows the patient to redefine their former and present conflicts and offers the opportunity for them to better comprehend their feelings and experiences and find healthy outlets for uncomfortable feelings. This is just one of the ways that therapy animals facilitate patient treatment and allow therapists to better understand different aspects of the patient's life. These insights arise from the interaction of the patient, the therapist, and the therapeutic animal.

Given the fact that therapy dogs are often the recipient of transference, the analyst has the time and space to have a clearer look at the patient's conflicts and internal unconscious processes. Patients are often encouraged to see the therapy dog (and therapist) as attachment figures and transitional objects (these being unconscious processes), allowing them to have the space and resources to explore unhealthy and/or cyclic intrapsychic processes. Of course, some patients may be resistant to bonding with the dog and/or the therapist and this response should be discussed in therapy. An additional benefit of animal-assisted psychoanalytic psychotherapy is that positive feelings towards the animal can help patients remain in treatment, even when things get challenging.

To exemplify the theoretical framework discussed in this chapter, a case of a woman who was helped by her therapy dog to begin her therapeutic process is included below.

Case Example

Maria is a 22-year-old patient who has been diagnosed with neurologic immaturity by a licensed neurologist. She is very functional and able to communicate verbally and in writing, and she has the ability to function in the social world with specific circles of people. She experiences a tremendous amount of negative self-talk, she constantly reminds herself that she has a disability, that she has less capabilities than every other person in her world, and therefore despises herself.

During her first sessions, Maria would avoid making eye contact. When a question was asked, she would nod her head indicating she was listening but would offer no response. From the first session, Maria showed particular interest in Kika, a dachshund therapy dog who was always part of the session. Maria would play with Kika, using her toys, telling her stories, and even singing her songs. One day she decided to start howling at Kika. Both Maria and Kika were surprised when, after a few sessions where Kika just listened curiously, she started howling back to Maria. They would howl back and forth for a long time during each session (see Video 36.1), and eventually Maria asked her therapist to join them, to also howl. As therapy continued, thanks to the acceptance that Kika showed, and the bonding they experienced through their "own language", Maria felt able to open up. She started by talking mainly about dogs, yet with time, she began sharing her feelings and thoughts about her life events.

Video 36.1

Kika, a dachshund therapy dog, howling with client Maria.

https://www.cabidigital library. org/ doi/ book/ 10.1079/9781800622616. 0000

Discussion Questions

1. How do you think howling with Kika helped Maria open up in therapy?
2. Do you think that patients like Maria are able to transfer their feelings of unconditional acceptance offered by a therapy dog to their therapist?

S. Smilovici

Index

Note: Page numbers in **bold** type refer to **figures;** page numbers in *italic* type refer to *tables*.

CABI – who we are and what we do

This book is published by **CABI**, an international not-for-profit organisation that improves people's lives worldwide by providing information and applying scientific expertise to solve problems in agriculture and the environment.

CABI is also a global publisher producing key scientific publications, including world renowned databases, as well as compendia, books, ebooks and full text electronic resources. We publish content in a wide range of subject areas including: agriculture and crop science / animal and veterinary sciences / ecology and conservation / environmental science / horticulture and plant sciences / human health, food science and nutrition / international development / leisure and tourism.

The profits from CABI's publishing activities enable us to work with farming communities around the world, supporting them as they battle with poor soil, invasive species and pests and diseases, to improve their livelihoods and help provide food for an ever growing population.

CABI is an international intergovernmental organisation, and we gratefully acknowledge the core financial support from our member countries (and lead agencies) including:

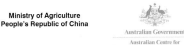
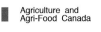

Discover more

To read more about CABI's work, please visit: **www.cabi.org**

Browse our books or explore our online products at **https://www.cabidigitallibrary.org**

Interested in writing for CABI? Find information for authors here: **https://www. cabidigitallibrary.org/books/authors**